First supplement to
McCance and Widdowson's
The Composition of Foods

Ministry of Agriculture, Fisheries and Food

Medical Research Council

First supplement to
McCance and Widdowson's
The Composition of Foods

Amino acids, mg per 100 g food
Fatty acids, g per 100 g food

By A. A. Paul, D. A. T. Southgate
and J. Russell

London
HER MAJESTY'S STATIONERY OFFICE

Amsterdam   New York   Oxford
ELSEVIER/NORTH-HOLLAND BIOMEDICAL PRESS

© *Crown copyright* 1980
First published 1980

Sole distributors outside the UK and Eire
Elsevier/North-Holland Biomedical Press
335 Jan van Gralenstraat, PO Box 211.
Amsterdam, The Netherlands

Sole distributors for the USA and Canada
Elsevier/North-Holland Inc.
52 Vanderbilt Avenue
New York, NY 10017, USA

Library of Congress Cataloging in Publication Data

Paul, A   A
 First supplement to McCance and Widdowson's The composition of foods.

 Bibliography: p.
 Includes index.
  1. Food-Composition. 2. Amino acids. 3. Acids, Fatty.
I. McCance, Robert Alexander, 1899–   *Composition of foods.*
II. Southgate, D. A. T., joint author. III. Russell, J., joint author.
IV. Title.
TX551.M13 1978 Suppl.   641.1   80-12283
ISBN 0-444-80220-7 (Elsevier/North-Holland)

Typographic design by HMSO

ISBN HMSO 0 11 450038 X
ISBN Elsevier/North-Holland 0 444 80220 7

Preface to the first supplement

In the 4th edition of McCance and Widdowson's 'The Composition of Foods' (Paul and Southgate 1978), amino acids and fatty acids are given, in sections 2 and 3, as mg/g nitrogen and g/100 g fatty acids respectively. This method enables the data to be presented in a concise form, as foods with the same amino acid or fatty acid composition can be given as a single entry. However, it is a straightforward procedure to calculate by computer the amino acid and fatty acid composition of each food given in Section I of the book, and this has accordingly been done for all foods where data are available. The following tables are intended as a supplement to 'The Composition of Foods', to which reference should be made for guidance on the description of samples, sources of the data, and the relevant cross references between the values in these tables and sections 1–3 of the tables in 'The Composition of Foods'.

A. A. Paul
MRC Dunn Nutrition Unit
Milton Road
Cambridge CB4 1XJ

D. A. T. Southgate
Food Research Institute
Colney Lane
Norwich

J. Russell
Ministry of Agriculture, Fisheries and Food
90–96 Cannon Street, London EC4N 6HT

May 1979

Contents

All the values in the tables are expressed in metric units; the imperial equivalents are as follows:

1 ounce (oz)	=	28.35 g	100 g	= 3.53 oz
1 pound (lb)	=	453.6 g	1 kg	= 2.2 lb (2 lb 3 oz)
1 pint (pt)	=	568 ml	1 litre	= 1.76 pt

Introduction

Method of calculation

The values for amino acids and fatty acids per 100 g food have been calculated as described on pages 348–9 of 'The Composition of Foods'. For convenience, these pages are repeated below.

Amino acids per 100 g are obtained by multiplying the total nitrogen (g/100 g, given in section 1) by the amino acids composition (mg amino acid per g N) of the appropriate item in section 2 of the fourth edition of 'The Composition of Foods'.

For example:

Item 252 **Beef rump steak** grilled, lean and fat
Total N = 4.36 g/100 g
Corresponding item in amino acid section, 2237

	Amino acids			
	Ile	Leu	Lys	etc
Amino acids in 2237 (mg/gN)	320	500	570	
Amino acids in 252 (mg/100 g)				
= (4.36 × values in 2237)	1395	2180	2485	etc

The values for cooked dishes are based on the information given in part 2 of Appendix 5 ('The Composition of Foods', 4th edition). The amino acids in the ingredients are multiplied by the amount of total nitrogen contributed by the ingredients to 100 g of the dish.

For example:

Item 116 **Pancakes**

Ingredients	Item in section 2	Total N contributed by ingredients
Flour	2011	0.43
Milk	2123	0.32
Egg	2165	0.25

The amino acids in the cooked dish are derived as follows:

	Amino acids			
	Ile	Leu	Lys	etc
From flour (0.43 × values in 2011)	103	189	52	
milk (0.32 × values in 2123)	112	205	163	
egg (0.25 × values in 2165)	88	130	98	
Amino acids in item 116 (mg/100 g) =	303	524	313	etc

Fatty acids per 100 g are calculated in a similar way using the compositions given in section 3, *except* that the factor giving the proportion of fatty acids in the total fat must also be used in the calculation (see p 17 of 'The Composition of Foods', 4th edition).

For example:

Item 252 **Beef rump steak** grilled, lean and fat
Fat 12.1 g/100 g; factor 0.935
Corresponding item in fatty acid section 3240

	Fatty acids			
	14:0	15:0	16:0	etc
Fatty acids in item 3240 (g/100 g total fatty acids)	3.2	0.6	26.9	
Fatty acids in item 252 (g/100 g) = (12.1 × 0.935 × values in 3240/100)	0.36	0.07	3.04	

For cooked dishes the values in the fatty acid section are multiplied by values for the fatty acids contributed by the ingredients of the dish.

For example:

Item 116 **Pancakes**

Ingredient	Item in section 3	Fat contributed	Factor
Flour	3008	0.29	0.70
Milk	3123	2.20	0.945
Eggs	3165	1.39	0.830
Lard	3185	12.42	0.956

The fatty acids in the cooked dish are derived as follows:

	Fatty acids		
	14:0	16:0	18:0
From flour (0.29 × 0.70 × values in 3008/100)	Tr	0.04	Tr
milk (2.20 × 0.945 × values in 3123/100)	0.23	0.54	0.23
eggs (1.39 × 0.830 × values in 3165/100)	Tr	0.33	0.11
lard (12.42 × 0.956 × values in 3185/100)	0.19	3.18	1.85
Fatty acids in 116 (g/100 g)	0.42	4.09	2.19

The calculation has been carried out for all food items listed in Appendix 5 of 'The Composition of Foods' for which a code number is given for use in the amino acid or fatty acid sections.

Fatty acids additional calculations

Estimated values
In section 3 of 'The Composition of Foods', 4th edition, in a small number of cases no information could be given for a particular fatty acid, and a dash showed these situations. For the present calculation, estimated values, based on the amounts in related foods, have been inserted onto the computer file and the results obtained are indicated in parenthesis.

Joint headings
In some fats and oils, and some meat and fish, values are given for the sum of two or more fatty acids in section 3, e.g. 20:4 + 20:5. For the present calculation, individual values have been assigned to each fatty acid.

Factor for calculating fatty acid content of fat

A factor has been used for each fatty acid code, and these are given in the table below. These are based on the factors given in table 5 (p. 17) of 'The Composition of Foods'.

Variations in fatty acid content

For a number of foods, marked 'a' in Appendix 5, no calculation is possible as the fatty acid content will depend on the fat used in cooking. In addition, for some foods, the fatty acid content will depend on variations in the fats used in manufacture. These are marked in the following tables and due attention should be taken in the interpretation of the data. Other variations are noted in section 3, to which reference should be made. For *margarine* in particular, the recipe calculations have been carried out using the fatty acid values for margarine and hard animal and vegetable fats (3188). Where other margarines are used, the fatty acid composition will be different.

Table *Factors for multiplying fat content of food by in calculation of fatty acids per 100 g food. Factor given for each fatty acid code.*

Code	Factor	Code	Factor	Code	Factor	Code	Factor
Cereals		**Fats & Oils**		3394	0.932	**Vegetables**	
3002	0.72	3140	0.945	3395	0.932	3562	0.80
3005	0.82	3183–		3396	0.932	3569	0.80
3008	0.70	3194	0.956	3399	0.80	3597	0.80
3017	0.94	3196	0.942	3404	0.80	3609	0.80
3019	0.85	3197–		3408	0.953	3620	0.80
3021	0.72	3206	0.956	3411	0.953	3634	0.80
3030	0.80			3425	0.953	3639	0.80
3033	0.80	**Meat**				3657	0.80
3058	0.95			**Fish**		3664	0.80
3060	0.72	3209	0.932			3669	0.80
3061	0.95	3240	0.935	3438	0.70		
3063	0.95	3269	0.935	3451	0.70	**Fruit**	
3064	0.95	3299	0.932	3458	0.70	3675	0.80
3066	0.72	3314	0.945	3461	0.70	3692	0.956
3067	0.95	3328	0.945	3466	0.70	3693	0.80
3068	0.95	3332	0.945	3471	0.70		
3069	0.95	3334	0.945	3474	0.70	**Nuts**	
3070	0.95	3336	0.945	3482	0.90	3822	0.956
3072	0.95	3340	0.945	3491	0.90	3826	0.956
3074	0.95	3350	0.945	3494	0.90	3828	0.956
3077	0.95	3356	0.561	3498	0.90	3830	0.956
3079	0.95	3358	0.789	3501	0.95	3832	0.942
3083	0.95	3360	0.789	3502	0.90	3835	0.956
3107	0.945	3364	0.747	3503	0.90	3838	0.956
3108	0.956	3366	0.747	3508	0.95	3839	0.956
Milk		3368	0.747	3510	0.90		
		3371	0.741	3513	0.90	**Chocolate Products**	
3123	0.945	3373	0.741	3517	0.70	3857	0.950
3137	0.945	3375	0.741	3526	0.70	3858	0.956
3138	0.956	3377	0.741	3532	0.70	3868	0.956
		3379	0.741	3535	0.70	3873	0.956
Eggs		3384	0.75	3537	0.70		
3165	0.83	3391	0.80	3550	0.70		

Errata in the 4th edition of 'The Composition of Foods'

A number of errata have come to light during the course of calculations; these are:

Section 3: fatty acid composition

Food code	Food	Fatty acids	
3063	**Biscuits, digestive** chocolate	22:1	for 1.6 *read* 1.0
3068	**Biscuits, sandwich**	20:1–20:5	for 1.4 *read* 1.0
3072	**Biscuits, wafers** filled	Other	for 10:0 *read* 8:0

Appendix 5: Key to the use of amino acid and fatty acid numbers
Part 1

Food Code	Food	Amino acids	Fatty acids
4	**Bemax**		for 3207 *read* 3008
Insert			
188	**Margarine** hard, animal and vegetable oils	2123	3188
189	Hard, vegetable oils only	2123	3189
190	Soft, animal and vegetable oils	2123	3190
191	Soft, vegetable oils only	2123	3191
192	Polyunsaturated	2123	3192
620–629	**Peas**		for 3621 *read* 3620

Part 2

Food code	Food	Section 2 code	Section 3 code	Fat contributed per 100 g
90	**Pastry, choux** cooked		3187	for 5.4 *read* 15.4
428	**Bolognese sauce**	for 2595 *read* 2594		
548	**Fish pie**	for 2638 *read* 2639		

Arrangement of the tables

Amino acids
The amino acids are given, by their customary abbreviations, in the same order as in Section 2 of 'The Composition of Foods'.

Fatty acids
A larger range of fatty acids is set out than appeared in Section 3 of 'The Composition of Foods'. Where a particular fatty acid that appears in one part of the table is not listed in another part this indicates that that particular fatty acid is not present in the food group. The three groups of fatty acids—saturated, mono-unsaturated and polyunsaturated—are spread over two pages. For most foods the saturated fatty acids appear on the first page and the mono- and polyunsaturated on the following page; however for fish the arrangement has had to be altered slightly to take into account the wide range of poly-unsaturated fatty acids present in that food group.

Reference   Paul, A. A. and Southgate, D. A. T. (1978) *McCance and Widdowson's 'The Composition of Foods'* 4th revised edition. London H.M. Stationery Office.

The tables

Section 2A
Amino acid composition

mg per 100 g food

Isoleucine	lle	Arginine	Arg
Leucine	Leu	Histidine	His
Lysine	Lys	Alanine	Ala
Methionine	Met	Aspartic acid	Asp
Cystine	Cys	Glutamic acid	Glu
Phenylalanine	Phe	Glycine	Gly
Tyrosine	Tyr	Proline	Pro
Threonine	Thr	Serine	Ser
Tryptophan	Trp		
Valine	Val		

N indicates no information available

Cereals and cereal products

Amino acids (mg per 100g food)

No	Food	Ile	Leu	Lys	Met	Cys	Phe	Tyr	Thr	Trp	Val	Arg	His	Ala	Asp	Glu	Gly	Pro	Ser
	Grains, flours and starches																		
2	**Barley** pearl, raw	300	570	220	140	190	430	260	280	140	420	410	180	350	470	1990	320	920	340
3	boiled	100	190	74	46	64	150	87	97	46	140	140	60	120	160	680	110	310	120
4	**Bemax**	950	1910	680	450	730	1270	860	770	320	1270	1320	590	1040	1410	7760	1140	3000	500
5	**Bran** wheat	470	920	610	220	380	580	450	490	180	690	1100	430	780	1140	2870	900	870	670
6	**Cornflour**	21	70	15	11	9	28	22	21	4	27	23	15	42	35	110	21	50	28
7	**Custard powder**	21	70	15	11	9	28	22	21	4	27	23	15	42	35	110	21	50	28
9	**Flour** wholemeal (100%)	480	950	340	230	360	630	430	380	160	630	660	290	520	700	3870	570	1490	750
10	brown (85%)	470	950	320	230	360	630	430	380	160	610	590	290	430	610	4550	450	1730	790
11	white (72%) breadmaking	480	870	240	200	320	590	320	340	140	540	440	260	380	540	4080	400	1560	690
12	household plain	410	760	210	170	280	520	280	290	120	460	380	220	330	460	3540	340	1360	600
13	self-raising	390	720	200	160	260	490	260	280	110	440	360	210	310	440	3360	330	1290	570
14	patent (40%)	450	830	230	190	300	570	300	320	130	510	420	250	360	510	3890	380	1490	660
15	**Macaroni** raw	580	1060	290	240	390	720	390	410	170	650	530	310	460	650	4970	480	1900	840
16	boiled	180	330	90	75	120	230	120	130	53	200	170	98	140	200	1550	150	590	260
17	**Oatmeal** raw	510	950	490	230	360	660	450	450	170	680	830	280	590	1020	2780	620	680	620
18	**Porridge**	58	110	55	26	41	74	50	50	19	77	94	31	67	120	310	70	77	70

Amino acids (mg per 100g food)

No	Food	Ile	Leu	Lys	Met	Cys	Phe	Tyr	Thr	Trp	Val	Arg	His	Ala	Asp	Glu	Gly	Pro	Ser
	Grains, flours and starches, contd																		
19	**Rice** polished raw	260	560	250	140	110	330	270	230	87	390	510	160	390	650	1310	290	320	320
20	boiled	89	190	85	48	37	110	93	78	30	130	170	56	130	220	440	100	110	110
21	**Rye** flour (100%)	310	550	290	130	170	390	170	290	98	420	410	200	380	630	2110	380	830	340
23	**Semolina** raw	450	820	220	190	300	560	300	320	130	510	410	240	360	510	3850	370	1480	660
24	**Soya** flour full fat	1810	3160	2580	520	650	2000	1290	1550	520	1940	2900	1030	1740	4710	7550	1680	2190	2060
25	low fat	2220	3890	3180	640	790	2460	1590	1910	640	2380	3570	1270	2140	5800	9290	2060	2700	2540
26	**Spaghetti** raw	570	1050	290	240	380	720	380	410	170	650	530	310	450	650	4920	480	1890	840
27	boiled	180	330	89	74	120	220	120	130	52	200	160	96	140	200	1520	150	590	260
28	canned in tomato sauce	72	130	36	30	48	90	48	51	21	81	66	39	57	81	620	60	240	110
	Bread and rolls																		
30	**Bread,** wholemeal	320	630	230	150	240	420	290	260	110	420	440	200	350	470	2580	380	1000	500
31	brown	330	660	220	160	250	440	300	270	110	420	410	200	300	420	3150	310	1200	550
32	hovis	360	710	240	170	270	480	320	290	120	460	440	220	320	460	3430	340	1310	600
33	white	340	620	170	140	220	420	220	240	98	380	310	180	270	380	2880	280	1110	490

Amino acids (mg per 100g food)

No	Food	Ile	Leu	Lys	Met	Cys	Phe	Tyr	Thr	Trp	Val	Arg	His	Ala	Asp	Glu	Gly	Pro	Ser
	Bread contd																		
34	white, fried	320	590	160	130	210	400	210	230	93	360	290	170	250	360	2740	270	1050	470
35	toasted	410	740	200	170	270	510	270	290	120	460	370	220	320	460	3480	340	1340	590
36	dried crumbs	490	890	240	200	330	610	330	350	140	550	450	260	390	550	4180	410	1600	710
37	currant	270	490	130	110	180	340	180	190	78	300	250	150	210	300	2310	220	890	390
38	malt	310	610	220	150	230	410	280	250	100	410	420	190	340	450	2500	370	960	480
39	soda	350	640	240	150	200	420	240	260	100	410	310	190	270	420	2700	260	1040	480
40	**Rolls** brown, crusty	420	850	280	200	320	570	380	340	140	550	530	260	380	550	4080	400	1560	710
41	soft	430	850	290	210	330	570	390	350	140	550	530	270	390	550	4140	410	1580	720
42	white, crusty	490	900	250	200	330	610	330	350	140	550	450	270	390	550	4200	410	1610	710
43	soft	410	730	210	170	280	520	280	290	120	460	380	220	330	460	3540	340	1360	600
44	starch reduced	1850	3400	930	770	1240	2320	1240	1310	540	2080	1700	1000	1470	2080	5900	1540	6100	2700
45	**Chapatis** made with fat	300	600	200	140	230	400	270	240	99	380	370	190	270	380	2870	280	1090	500
46	made without fat	270	540	180	130	210	360	240	220	90	350	330	170	240	350	2590	260	990	450
	Breakfast cereals																		
47	**All-bran**	500	980	650	240	410	620	480	530	190	740	1180	460	840	1220	3070	960	940	720
48	**Cornflakes**	320	1080	240	170	140	430	330	320	55	410	360	240	650	540	1630	320	770	430
49	**Grapenuts**	410	730	300	190	260	590	350	390	190	570	560	240	480	650	2720	440	1260	460
50	**Muesli**	530	1000	510	240	380	690	460	460	180	710	860	290	620	1060	2900	640	710	640
51	**Puffed Wheat**	510	1030	370	240	390	680	460	420	170	680	710	320	560	760	4170	610	1610	810
52	**Ready Brek**	510	950	490	230	360	660	450	450	170	680	830	280	590	1020	2780	620	680	620
53	**Rice Krispies**	240	510	230	130	99	300	250	210	79	360	470	150	360	590	1190	270	290	290

Cereals and cereal products *continued*

No	Food	Ile	Leu	Lys	Met	Cys	Phe	Tyr	Thr	Trp	Val	Arg	His	Ala	Asp	Glu	Gly	Pro	Ser
	Breakfast cereals contd																		
54	**Shredded Wheat**	380	760	270	180	290	510	340	310	130	510	530	240	420	560	3100	450	1200	600
56	**Sugar Puffs**	210	420	150	100	160	280	190	170	71	280	290	130	230	310	1730	250	670	330
57	**Weetabix**	410	820	290	200	310	550	370	330	140	550	570	260	450	610	3350	490	1290	650
	Biscuits																		
58	**Chocolate** full coated	240	440	120	100	160	300	160	170	70	270	220	130	190	270	2060	200	790	350
59	**Cream crackers**	400	730	200	170	270	500	270	280	120	450	370	220	320	450	3420	330	1310	580
60	**Crispbread** rye	350	630	340	150	190	450	190	340	110	480	470	230	440	730	2430	440	950	390
61	wheat starch reduced	1910	3490	950	790	1270	2380	1270	1350	560	2140	1750	1030	1510	2140	6360	1590	6270	2780
62	**Digestive** plain	350	710	240	170	270	470	320	290	120	450	440	220	320	450	3390	340	1290	590
64	**Ginger nuts**	240	430	120	98	160	290	160	170	69	270	220	130	190	270	2020	200	770	340
65	**Home made**	290	510	200	140	160	340	200	220	87	350	280	150	250	400	1950	220	740	420
66	**Matzo**	440	810	220	190	300	560	300	320	130	500	410	240	350	500	3810	370	1460	650
67	**Oatcakes**	410	770	390	190	290	530	360	360	140	550	670	220	480	820	2240	500	550	500
68	**Sandwich**	210	380	100	87	140	260	140	150	61	240	190	110	170	240	1790	170	690	310
69	**Semi-sweet**	280	520	140	120	190	350	190	200	83	320	260	150	220	320	2430	240	930	410
70	**Short-sweet**	260	480	130	110	170	320	170	180	76	290	240	140	210	290	2230	220	850	380
71	**Shortbread**	260	480	140	110	170	330	180	190	76	300	240	140	210	300	2210	220	850	380
72	**Wafers** filled	200	360	98	82	130	250	130	140	57	220	180	110	160	220	1690	160	650	290
73	**Water biscuits**	450	830	230	190	300	570	300	320	130	510	420	250	360	510	3890	380	1490	660

Cereals and cereal products *continued*

No	Food	Ile	Leu	Lys	Met	Cys	Phe	Tyr	Thr	Trp	Val	Arg	His	Ala	Asp	Glu	Gly	Pro	Ser
	Cakes																		
74	**Fancy iced cakes**	160	250	79	66	110	200	110	110	46	180	150	86	130	180	1360	130	520	230
75	**Fruitcake** rich	150	250	140	99	80	170	110	140	47	200	200	98	160	320	880	120	290	240
76	rich iced	170	290	150	97	81	200	130	150	50	240	310	110	190	400	950	170	280	240
78	**Gingerbread**	270	460	210	130	140	300	190	210	79	320	260	140	230	380	1630	190	620	380
79	**Madeira cake**	230	410	110	94	150	280	150	160	66	250	210	120	180	250	1940	190	740	330
80	**Rock cakes**	240	410	180	120	130	270	170	190	71	290	250	130	210	360	1590	180	590	350
81	**Spongecake** with fat	320	510	280	160	140	330	220	270	97	400	320	150	290	510	1440	210	530	450
82	without fat	520	810	510	280	210	520	370	450	160	670	540	240	480	900	1890	320	670	730
	Buns and pastries																		
84	**Currant buns**	310	570	160	130	210	390	210	220	91	350	290	170	250	350	2680	260	1030	460
85	**Doughnuts**	250	450	120	100	170	310	170	180	72	280	230	130	200	280	2120	210	810	360
86	**Eclairs**	210	350	210	110	91	230	150	190	66	280	230	100	200	370	980	150	350	290
87	**Jam tarts**	140	260	76	58	90	170	94	100	42	160	130	78	120	230	1170	120	450	210
88	**Mince pies**	170	310	90	78	120	220	120	130	50	200	170	100	140	220	1490	150	560	260

Cereals and cereal products *continued*

Amino acids (mg per 100g food)

No	Food	Ile	Leu	Lys	Met	Cys	Phe	Tyr	Thr	Trp	Val	Arg	His	Ala	Asp	Glu	Gly	Pro	Ser
	Buns and pastries contd																		
89	**Pastry, choux** raw	280	440	240	140	120	290	190	230	84	350	280	130	250	440	1250	180	460	390
90	cooked	420	690	380	220	190	440	300	360	130	540	430	200	380	690	1930	280	700	600
91	**flaky** raw	190	340	92	77	120	230	120	130	54	210	170	100	150	210	1590	150	610	270
92	cooked	250	450	120	100	160	310	160	170	71	280	220	130	190	280	2100	200	810	360
93	**shortcrust** raw	250	450	120	100	170	310	170	180	72	280	230	130	200	280	2120	210	810	360
94	cooked	290	530	140	120	190	360	190	200	84	320	260	160	230	320	2470	240	950	420
95	**Scones**	330	610	230	150	190	400	230	250	95	390	290	180	260	400	2550	250	990	460
96	**Scotch pancakes**	320	560	280	150	150	350	230	250	92	390	290	160	260	440	1930	210	740	430
	Puddings																		
97	**Apple crumble**	76	140	46	31	49	92	49	56	22	86	69	41	64	120	620	65	240	110
98	**Bread and butter pudding**	330	560	400	170	93	320	250	290	93	430	290	170	270	540	1270	170	480	410
99	**Cheesecake**	210	360	220	110	78	220	160	180	61	270	190	110	180	330	1000	120	380	280
100	**Christmas pudding**	210	370	170	120	120	250	160	180	65	280	290	130	210	410	1370	180	470	320
101	**Custard** egg	320	540	420	170	74	300	240	290	90	420	280	160	260	540	1040	150	400	380
102	made with powder	210	380	310	110	36	200	170	190	54	280	150	110	140	320	860	84	350	220
103	**Custard tart**	280	500	270	140	120	310	200	230	81	350	250	150	230	410	1580	180	600	370
104	**Dumpling**	120	220	61	51	82	150	82	87	36	140	110	66	97	140	1050	100	400	180

No	Fcod	Ile	Leu	Lys	Met	Cys	Phe	Tyr	Thr	Trp	Val	Arg	His	Ala	Asp	Glu	Gly	Pro	Ser
	Puddings contd																		
106	**Fruit pie** with pastry top	80	150	56	31	50	94	50	61	23	91	72	44	70	150	620	70	230	110
107	**Ice cream** dairy	200	370	300	100	35	200	160	180	52	270	150	110	140	310	840	81	340	220
108	non-dairy	180	330	270	94	31	180	150	160	47	240	130	99	130	280	750	73	310	190
109	**Jelly** packet, cubes	99	200	280	55	0	140	22	130	0	150	540	44	670	410	690	1660	950	250
110	made with water	23	45	63	13	0	33	5	30	0	35	120	10	150	93	160	380	220	58
111	made with milk	100	190	180	52	13	110	67	98	20	140	180	52	210	210	470	410	350	140
112	**Lemon meringue pie**	220	360	190	110	100	230	150	180	67	280	220	110	200	350	1060	150	390	310
113	**Meringues**	300	430	310	190	94	310	210	260	94	420	290	120	310	580	650	170	210	390
114	**Milk pudding**	220	410	310	110	43	220	180	200	59	300	190	120	170	360	930	100	360	240
115	canned, rice	220	410	310	110	43	220	180	200	59	300	190	120	170	360	930	100	360	240
116	**Pancakes**	300	520	310	150	120	320	220	250	86	380	270	150	240	450	1530	180	580	390
117	**Queen of puddings**	250	420	290	140	79	250	190	220	74	330	240	120	220	430	930	140	350	330
118	**Sponge pudding** steamed	280	470	230	140	140	310	200	230	84	350	270	140	240	420	1560	190	590	400
119	**Suet pudding** steamed	200	370	160	90	110	240	140	150	57	240	170	110	150	250	1490	140	580	270
120	**Treacle tart**	160	290	78	65	100	200	100	110	46	180	140	85	120	180	1340	130	510	230
121	**Trifle**	180	320	230	95	50	180	140	160	51	240	170	95	150	320	740	99	280	220
122	**Yorkshire pudding**	340	590	350	170	130	360	250	280	97	430	300	170	270	510	1720	200	660	440

Milk and milk products

Amino acids (mg per 100g food)

No	Food	Ile	Leu	Lys	Met	Cys	Phe	Tyr	Thr	Trp	Val	Arg	His	Ala	Asp	Glu	Gly	Pro	Ser
	Milk, cows'																		
124	fresh, whole summer	180	330	270	94	31	180	150	160	47	240	130	99	130	280	750	73	310	190
125	winter	180	330	270	94	31	180	150	160	47	240	130	99	130	280	750	73	310	190
127	fresh, whole, Channel Isles summer	200	360	290	100	34	190	160	170	50	260	140	110	130	300	810	78	330	210
128	winter	200	360	290	100	34	190	160	170	50	260	140	110	130	300	810	78	330	210
129	sterilized	180	330	270	94	31	180	150	160	47	240	130	99	130	280	750	73	310	190
130	longlife (UHT treated)	180	330	270	94	31	180	150	160	47	240	130	99	130	280	750	73	310	190
131	fresh skimmed	190	340	270	95	32	180	150	160	48	240	130	100	130	280	760	74	310	200
132	condensed, whole, sweetened	460	830	660	230	78	440	360	400	120	600	330	250	310	690	1870	180	770	480
133	condensed, skimmed, sweetened	540	990	790	280	93	530	430	480	140	710	390	300	370	820	2230	220	920	570
134	evaporated, whole, unsweetened	470	860	690	240	81	460	380	420	120	620	340	260	320	720	1940	190	800	500
135	dried, whole	1440	2640	2100	740	250	1400	1150	1280	370	1900	1030	780	990	2180	5930	580	2430	1520
136	dried, skimmed	2000	3650	2910	1030	340	1940	1600	1770	510	2620	1430	1080	1370	3020	8210	800	3360	2110
138	**Milk, human** mature	64	120	86	18	24	46	36	54	28	82	46	30	50	110	210	30	120	52
139	transitional	99	180	130	28	37	71	56	84	43	130	71	47	78	170	330	47	180	81
140	**Butter** salted	25	45	36	13	4	24	20	22	6	32	18	13	17	37	100	10	41	26

No	Food	Ile	Leu	Lys	Met	Cys	Phe	Tyr	Thr	Trp	Val	Arg	His	Ala	Asp	Glu	Gly	Pro	Ser
	Cream																		
142	single summer	130	240	190	68	23	130	110	120	34	180	95	72	91	200	550	53	220	140
143	winter	130	240	190	68	23	130	110	120	34	180	95	72	91	200	550	53	220	140
145	double summer	84	150	120	43	14	82	67	74	22	110	60	46	58	130	350	34	140	89
146	winter	84	150	120	43	14	82	67	74	22	110	60	46	58	130	350	34	140	89
148	whipping summer	110	190	150	54	18	100	84	93	27	140	75	57	72	160	430	42	180	110
149	winter	110	190	150	54	18	100	84	93	27	140	75	57	72	160	430	42	180	110
150	sterilized canned	140	260	200	72	24	140	110	120	36	180	100	76	96	210	580	56	240	150
	Cheese																		
151	Camembert type	1250	2290	1830	640	220	1220	1000	1110	320	1650	900	680	860	1900	5160	500	2110	1330
152	Cheddar type	1430	2610	2080	730	250	1390	1140	1270	370	1880	1020	780	980	2160	5880	570	2410	1510
153	Danish Blue type	1260	2310	1840	650	220	1230	1010	1120	330	1660	900	690	870	1910	5200	510	2130	1340
154	Edam type	1340	2450	1950	690	230	1300	1070	1180	340	1760	960	730	920	2030	5500	540	2250	1410
155	Parmesan	1930	3520	2810	990	330	1870	1540	1710	500	2530	1380	1050	1320	2920	7920	770	3250	2040
156	Stilton	1410	2570	2050	720	240	1370	1130	1250	360	1850	1010	760	970	2130	5790	560	2370	1490
157	Cottage cheese	750	1370	1090	390	130	730	600	660	190	980	540	410	510	1130	3080	300	1260	790
158	Cream cheese	170	310	250	88	29	170	140	150	44	230	120	93	120	260	710	69	290	180
159	Processed cheese	1180	2150	1720	610	200	1150	940	1050	300	1550	840	640	810	1790	4850	470	1990	1250
160	Cheese spread	1010	1840	1460	520	170	980	800	890	260	1320	720	550	690	1520	4130	400	1690	1060
	Yogurt low fat																		
161	natural	300	560	340	100	39	290	240	220	62	340	140	160	190	340	900	130	370	280
162	flavoured	310	570	340	100	40	290	250	220	63	340	140	170	190	340	910	130	380	280
163	fruit	300	550	330	99	38	280	240	210	61	330	140	160	180	330	870	120	370	270
164	hazelnut	320	530	350	110	41	300	250	230	66	350	150	170	200	350	940	130	390	300

No	Food	Ile	Leu	Lys	Met	Cys	Phe	Tyr	Thr	Trp	Val	Arg	His	Ala	Asp	Glu	Gly	Pro	Ser
	Eggs																		
165	whole, raw	690	1020	770	390	220	630	490	630	220	930	750	300	670	1320	1480	370	470	970
166	white, raw	500	730	520	320	160	520	360	430	160	710	490	200	520	980	1090	290	360	660
167	yolk, raw	930	1370	1160	410	260	650	650	900	280	1110	1160	410	800	1700	1750	440	570	1390
168	dried	2440	3620	2720	1390	770	2230	1740	2230	770	3280	2650	1050	2370	4670	5230	1320	1670	3420
169	boiled	690	1020	770	390	220	630	490	630	220	930	750	300	670	1320	1480	370	470	970
170	fried	790	1180	880	450	250	720	570	720	250	1060	860	340	770	1510	1700	430	540	1110
171	poached	700	1040	780	400	220	640	500	640	220	940	760	300	680	1330	1490	380	480	980
172	omelette	580	860	650	330	180	530	410	530	180	780	630	250	560	1100	1240	310	400	810
173	scrambled	590	880	660	330	180	540	420	530	180	780	620	250	560	1110	1310	310	430	810
	Egg and cheese dishes																		
174	**Cauliflower cheese**	300	530	410	150	49	280	220	260	80	390	230	160	260	460	1170	180	450	270
175	**Cheese pudding**	550	960	710	290	140	540	420	490	150	720	460	280	430	890	2130	260	830	660
176	**Cheese soufflé**	610	1030	770	320	160	590	460	540	170	800	530	300	490	1000	2180	290	840	740
177	**Macaroni cheese**	380	690	470	190	110	390	290	320	100	480	290	210	270	540	1940	190	770	430
178	**Pizza**, cheese and tomato	470	850	570	230	140	490	360	400	130	590	370	260	350	690	2420	250	970	550
179	**Quiche Lorraine**	760	1290	1010	390	210	740	570	660	200	940	710`	420	660	1220	3170	480	1200	860
180	**Scotch egg**	560	860	700	300	210	530	370	500	170	700	670	290	630	1030	1950	580	770	700
181	**Welsh rarebit**	810	1480	1040	400	210	830	630	690	210	1040	610	440	570	1170	3970	390	1600	910

Fats and oils

Amino acids (mg per 100g food)

No	Food	Ile	Leu	Lys	Met	Cys	Phe	Tyr	Thr	Trp	Val	Arg	His	Ala	Asp	Glu	Gly	Pro	Ser
140	**Butter** salted	25	45	36	13	4	24	20	22	6	32	18	13	17	37	100	10	41	26
187	**Margarine** all kinds	7	13	10	4	1	7	6	6	2	9	5	4	5	11	29	3	12	7

Meat and meat products

Amino acids (mg per 100 g food)

No	Food	Ile	Leu	Lys	Met	Cys	Phe	Tyr	Thr	Trp	Val	Arg	His	Ala	Asp	Glu	Gly	Pro	Ser
	Bacon																		
208	**dressed carcase raw**	620	960	1100	330	170	560	460	560	150	670	830	420	790	1170	2120	690	670	540
210	**lean** average, raw	970	1490	1710	520	260	870	710	870	230	1030	1290	650	1230	1810	3300	1070	1030	840
211	**fat** average, raw	230	350	400	120	61	210	170	210	53	240	300	150	290	430	780	250	240	200
212	cooked	440	680	780	240	120	400	330	400	100	470	590	300	560	830	1510	490	470	390
213	**collar joint** raw, lean and fat	700	1080	1240	370	190	630	520	630	160	750	940	470	890	1310	2390	770	750	610
214	boiled, lean and fat	980	1500	1730	520	260	880	720	880	230	1040	1300	650	1240	1830	3330	1080	1040	850
215	lean only	1250	1910	2210	670	330	1120	920	1120	290	1330	1660	830	1580	2330	4240	1370	1330	1080
216	**gammon joint** raw, lean and fat	850	1300	1500	450	230	760	620	760	200	900	1130	560	1070	1580	2880	930	900	730
217	boiled, lean and fat	1190	1820	2090	630	320	1070	870	1070	280	1260	1580	790	1500	2210	4030	1300	1260	1030
218	lean only	1410	2160	2490	750	380	1270	1030	1270	330	1500	1880	940	1790	2630	4790	1550	1500	1220
219	**gammon rashers** grilled, lean and fat	1420	2170	2500	760	380	1270	1040	1270	330	1510	1890	940	1790	2640	4810	1560	1510	1230
220	lean only	1510	2310	2660	800	400	1360	1100	1360	350	1610	2010	1000	1910	2810	5120	1660	1610	1310
221	**rashers, raw** back, lean and fat	680	1040	1200	360	180	610	500	610	160	730	910	450	860	1270	2320	750	730	590
222	middle, lean and fat	680	1050	1210	370	180	620	500	620	160	730	910	460	870	1280	2330	750	730	590
223	streaky, lean and fat	700	1080	1240	370	190	630	520	630	160	750	940	470	890	1310	2390	770	750	610
225	**rashers, fried** average, lean only	1570	2410	2780	840	420	1420	1150	1420	370	1680	2100	1050	1990	2930	5350	1730	1680	1360
226	back, lean and fat	1200	1840	2120	640	320	1080	880	1080	280	1280	1600	800	1520	2230	4070	1320	1280	1040
227	middle, lean and fat	1160	1780	2050	620	310	1040	850	1040	270	1240	1540	770	1470	2160	3940	1270	1240	1000
228	streaky, lean and fat	1110	1700	1960	590	300	1000	810	1000	260	1180	1480	740	1400	2070	3760	1220	1180	960
230	**rashers, grilled** average, lean only	1460	2250	2590	780	390	1320	1070	1320	340	1560	1950	980	1850	2730	4980	1610	1560	1270
231	back, lean and fat	1210	1860	2140	650	320	1090	890	1090	280	1290	1620	810	1540	2260	4120	1330	1290	1050
232	middle, lean and fat	1190	1830	2110	640	320	1080	880	1080	280	1270	1590	800	1510	2230	4060	1310	1270	1040
233	streaky, lean and fat	1180	1800	2080	630	310	1060	860	1060	270	1250	1570	780	1490	2200	4000	1290	1250	1020

Amino acids (mg per 100 g food)

No	Fcod	Ile	Leu	Lys	Met	Cys	Phe	Tyr	Thr	Trp	Val	Arg	His	Ala	Asp	Glu	Gly	Pro	Ser
	Beef																		
235	**dressed carcase** raw	810	1270	1440	430	200	710	610	730	200	840	1060	580	1010	1520	2730	890	810	710
237	**lean**, average, raw	1040	1630	1850	550	260	910	780	940	260	1070	1370	750	1300	1950	3510	1140	1040	910
240	**fat**, average, raw	450	700	800	240	110	390	340	410	110	460	590	320	560	840	1510	490	450	390
241	cooked	610	960	1090	330	150	540	460	550	150	630	800	440	760	1150	2060	670	610	540
242	**brisket** raw, lean and fat	860	1340	1530	460	210	750	640	780	210	880	1130	620	1070	1610	2890	940	860	750
243	boiled, lean and fat	1410	2210	2510	750	350	1240	1063	1280	350	1460	1850	1010	1760	2650	4760	1540	1410	1240
244	**forerib** raw, lean and fat	820	1280	1460	440	210	720	610	740	210	850	1080	590	1020	1540	2770	900	820	720
245	roast, lean and fat	1150	1800	2050	610	290	1010	860	1040	290	1190	1510	830	1440	2150	3880	1260	1150	1010
246	lean only	1430	2230	2540	760	360	1250	1070	1290	360	1470	1870	1030	1780	2680	4820	1560	1430	1250
247	**mince** raw	960	1510	1720	510	240	840	720	870	240	990	1260	690	1200	1810	3250	1050	960	840
248	stewed	1180	1850	2100	630	300	1030	890	1070	300	1220	1550	850	1480	2210	3990	1290	1180	1030
249	**rump steak** raw, lean and fat	970	1510	1720	510	240	850	730	880	240	1000	1270	700	1210	1810	3260	1060	970	850
250	fried, lean and fat	1470	2290	2610	780	370	1280	1100	1330	370	1510	1920	1050	1830	2750	4950	1600	1470	1280
251	lean only	1570	2460	2800	840	390	1380	1180	1430	390	1620	2070	1130	1970	2950	5310	1720	1570	1380
252	grilled, lean and fat	1400	2180	2490	740	350	1220	1050	1260	350	1440	1830	1000	1740	2620	4710	1530	1400	1220
253	lean only	1470	2290	2610	780	370	1280	1100	1330	370	1510	1920	1050	1830	2750	4950	1600	1470	1280
254	**silverside** salted, boiled, lean and fat	1470	2290	2610	780	370	1280	1100	1330	370	1510	1920	1050	1830	2750	4950	1600	1470	1280
255	lean only	1650	2580	2940	880	410	1450	1240	1500	410	1700	2170	1190	2060	3100	5570	1810	1650	1450
256	**sirloin** raw, lean and fat	850	1330	1510	450	210	740	640	770	210	880	1110	610	1060	1590	2860	930	850	740
257	roast, lean and fat	1210	1890	2150	640	300	1060	910	1090	300	1240	1580	870	1513	2260	4070	1320	1210	1060
258	lean only	1410	2210	2510	750	350	1240	1060	1280	350	1460	1850	1010	1760	2650	4760	1540	1410	1240
259	**stewing steak** raw, lean and fat	1030	1620	1840	550	260	900	780	940	260	1070	1360	740	1290	1940	3490	1130	1030	900
260	stewed, lean and fat	1580	2470	2820	840	400	1380	1190	1430	400	1630	2080	1140	1980	2960	5340	1730	1580	1380
261	**topside** raw, lean and fat	1000	1570	1780	530	250	880	750	910	250	1030	1320	720	1250	1880	3380	1100	1000	880
262	roast, lean and fat	1360	2130	2430	720	340	1190	1020	1240	340	1410	1790	980	1700	2560	4600	1490	1360	1190
263	lean only	1490	2340	2660	790	370	1310	1120	1350	370	1540	1960	1070	1870	2800	5040	1640	1490	1310

Meat and meat products *continued*

Amino acids (mg per 100 g food)

Lamb

No	Food	Ile	Leu	Lys	Met	Cys	Phe	Tyr	Thr	Trp	Val	Arg	His	Ala	Asp	Glu	Gly	Pro	Ser
264	**dressed carcase** raw	680	1050	1430	370	190	560	520	680	190	700	890	470	840	1330	2460	730	680	630
266	**lean** average, raw	970	1500	2030	530	270	800	730	970	270	1000	1270	670	1200	1900	3500	1030	970	900
269	**fat** average, raw	290	450	600	160	79	240	220	290	79	300	380	200	360	560	1040	310	290	270
270	cooked	530	820	1100	290	150	430	400	530	150	540	690	360	650	1030	1900	560	530	490
271	**breast** raw, lean and fat	770	1200	1630	430	210	640	590	770	210	800	1020	530	960	1520	2800	830	770	720
272	roast, lean and fat	890	1370	1860	490	240	730	670	890	240	920	1160	610	1100	1740	3200	950	890	820
273	lean only	1190	1840	2500	650	330	980	900	1190	330	1230	1550	820	1470	2330	4300	1270	1190	1100
274	**chops, loin** raw, lean and fat	680	1050	1430	370	190	560	520	680	190	700	890	470	840	1330	2460	730	680	630
275	grilled, lean and fat	1090	1690	2290	600	300	900	830	1090	300	1130	1430	750	1350	2140	3950	1170	1090	1020
276	lean and fat (weighed with bone)	850	1320	1790	470	230	700	650	850	230	880	1110	590	1060	1670	3080	910	850	790
277	lean only	1290	2000	2710	710	360	1070	980	1290	360	1330	1690	890	1600	2530	4660	1380	1290	1200
278	lean only (weighed with fat and bone)	710	1100	1490	390	200	590	540	710	200	730	930	490	880	1390	2560	760	710	660
279	**cutlets** raw, lean and fat	680	1060	1430	380	190	560	520	680	190	710	890	470	850	1340	2470	730	680	640
280	grilled, lean and fat	1070	1660	2250	590	290	880	810	1070	290	1100	1400	740	1330	2100	3860	1140	1070	990
281	lean and fat (weighed with bone)	710	1090	1480	390	190	580	540	710	190	730	920	490	880	1390	2550	750	710	660
282	lean only	1290	2000	2710	710	360	1070	980	1290	360	1330	1690	890	1600	2530	4660	1380	1290	1200
283	lean only (weighed with fat and bone)	570	880	1190	310	160	470	430	570	160	590	740	390	700	1110	2050	610	570	530
284	**leg** raw, lean and fat	830	1290	1750	460	230	690	630	830	230	860	1090	570	1030	1630	3000	890	830	770
285	roast, lean and fat	1210	1880	2550	670	330	1000	920	1210	330	1250	1590	840	1510	2380	4390	1300	1210	1130
286	lean only	1370	2120	2870	750	380	1130	1040	1370	380	1410	1790	940	1700	2690	4950	1460	1370	1270
287	**scrag and neck** raw, lean and fat	730	1130	1530	400	200	600	550	730	200	750	950	500	900	1430	2630	780	730	680
288	stewed, lean and fat	1190	1850	2500	660	330	980	900	1190	330	1230	1560	820	1480	2340	4310	1270	1190	1110
289	lean only	1290	2000	2710	710	360	1070	980	1290	360	1330	1690	890	1600	2530	4660	1380	1290	1200
290	lean only (weighed with fat and bone)	660	1020	1380	360	180	540	500	660	180	680	860	450	810	1290	2370	700	660	610

Meat and meat products *continued*

No	Food	Ile	Leu	Lys	Met	Cys	Phe	Tyr	Thr	Trp	Val	Arg	His	Ala	Asp	Glu	Gly	Pro	Ser
	Lamb *cont*																		
291	**shoulder** raw, lean and fat	730	1130	1530	400	200	600	550	730	200	750	950	500	900	1430	2630	780	730	680
292	roast, lean and fat	920	1430	1940	510	250	760	700	920	250	950	1210	640	1150	1810	3340	990	920	860
293	lean only	1100	1710	2320	610	300	910	840	1100	300	1140	1440	760	1370	2170	3990	1180	1100	1030
	Pork																		
294	**dressed carcase** raw	610	960	1310	370	170	520	500	590	150	650	810	590	740	1220	2180	720	650	570
296	**lean** average, raw	920	1450	1970	560	260	790	760	890	230	990	1220	890	1120	1840	3290	1090	990	860
299	**fat** average, raw	300	480	650	180	80	260	250	290	76	320	400	290	370	610	1080	360	320	280
300	cooked	660	1040	1420	400	190	570	550	640	170	710	880	640	810	1330	2370	780	710	620
301	**belly, rashers** raw, lean and fat	680	1070	1460	420	200	590	560	660	170	730	900	660	830	1370	2440	810	730	630
302	grilled, lean and fat	950	1490	2030	580	270	810	780	910	240	1010	1250	910	1150	1890	3380	1120	1010	880
303	**chops, loin** raw, lean and fat	710	1120	1530	430	200	610	590	690	180	770	940	690	870	1430	2550	840	770	660
304	grilled, lean and fat	1270	2000	2730	770	360	1090	1050	1230	320	1370	1680	1230	1550	2550	4550	1500	1370	1180
305	lean and fat (weighed with bone)	990	1560	2130	600	280	850	820	960	250	1070	1310	960	1210	1990	3550	1170	1070	920
306	lean only	1450	2280	3100	880	410	1240	1190	1400	360	1550	1910	1400	1760	2900	5170	1710	1550	1340
307	lean only (weighed with fat and bone)	850	1340	1830	520	240	730	700	820	210	920	1130	820	1040	1710	3050	1010	920	790
308	**leg** raw, lean and fat	750	1170	1600	450	210	640	610	720	190	800	980	720	900	1490	2660	880	800	690
309	roast, lean and fat	1200	1890	2580	730	340	1030	990	1160	300	1290	1590	1160	1460	2410	4300	1420	1290	1120
310	lean only	1380	2160	2950	840	390	1180	1130	1330	340	1470	1820	1330	1670	2750	4910	1620	1470	1280
	Veal																		
311	**cutlet** fried	1610	2510	2860	850	400	1410	1210	1460	400	1660	2110	1160	2010	3010	5420	1760	1610	1410
312	**fillet** raw	1080	1690	1920	570	270	940	810	980	270	1110	1420	780	1350	2020	3640	1180	1080	940
313	roast	1620	2530	2880	860	400	1410	1210	1470	400	1670	2120	1160	2020	3030	5450	1770	1620	1410

Meat and meat products *continued*

Amino acids (mg per 100 g food)

No	Food	Ile	Leu	Lys	Met	Cys	Phe	Tyr	Thr	Trp	Val	Arg	His	Ala	Asp	Glu	Gly	Pro	Ser
	Poultry and game																		
314	**Chicken** raw, meat only	950	1540	1840	490	260	920	720	850	230	980	1280	620	1180	1870	3380	1020	850	820
315	meat and skin	820	1330	1580	420	230	790	620	730	200	850	1100	540	1020	1610	2910	870	730	710
316	light meat	1010	1640	1950	520	280	980	770	910	240	1050	1360	660	1260	1990	3600	1080	910	870
317	dark meat	890	1440	1710	460	250	860	670	800	210	920	1190	580	1100	1740	3150	950	800	770
318	boiled, meat only	1350	2200	2620	700	370	1310	1030	1210	330	1400	1820	890	1680	2660	4810	1450	1210	1170
319	light meat	1380	2230	2660	710	380	1330	1050	1240	330	1430	1850	900	1710	2710	4890	1470	1240	1190
320	dark meat	1330	2150	2570	690	370	1280	1010	1190	320	1370	1790	870	1650	2610	4720	1420	1190	1150
321	roast, meat only	1150	1870	2220	600	320	1110	870	1030	280	1190	1550	750	1430	2260	4090	1230	1030	990
322	meat and skin	1050	1700	2020	540	290	1010	790	940	250	1080	1410	690	1300	2060	3720	1120	940	900
323	light meat	1230	1990	2370	640	340	1190	930	1100	300	1270	1650	810	1530	2420	4370	1310	1100	1060
324	dark meat	1070	1730	2070	550	300	1030	810	960	260	1110	1440	700	1330	2100	3800	1140	960	920
325	wing quarter (weighed with bone)																		
326	leg quarter (weighed with bone)	580	940	1110	300	160	560	440	520	140	600	780	380	720	1130	2050	620	520	500
327	**Duck** raw, meat only	980	1540	1730	540	250	880	730	880	250	1010	1320	500	1200	1830	3280	1010	980	820
328	meat, fat and skin	560	880	990	310	140	500	410	500	140	580	760	290	680	1040	1870	580	560	470
329	roast, meat only	1260	1990	2230	690	320	1130	930	1130	320	1300	1700	650	1540	2350	4210	1300	1260	1050
330	meat, fat and skin	970	1540	1730	530	250	880	720	880	250	1010	1320	500	1190	1820	3270	1010	970	820
331	**Goose** roast	1450	2300	2580	800	380	1310	1080	1310	380	1500	1970	750	1780	2720	4880	1500	1450	1220
332	**Grouse** roast	1550	2450	2750	850	400	1400	1150	1400	400	1600	2100	800	1900	2900	5200	1600	1550	1300
333	roast (weighed with bone)	1020	1620	1820	560	260	920	760	920	260	1060	1390	530	1250	1910	3430	1060	1020	860
334	**Partridge** roast	1820	2880	3230	1000	470	1640	1350	1640	470	1880	2470	940	2230	3410	6110	1880	1820	1530
335	roast (weighed with bone)	1090	1730	1940	600	280	990	810	990	280	1130	1480	560	1340	2040	3660	1130	1090	920

Meat and meat products *continued*

Amino acids (mg per 100 g food)

Poultry and game *contd*

No	Food	Ile	Leu	Lys	Met	Cys	Phe	Tyr	Thr	Trp	Val	Arg	His	Ala	Asp	Glu	Gly	Pro	Ser
336	**Pheasant** roast	1600	2520	2830	880	410	1440	1190	1440	410	1650	2160	820	1960	2990	5360	1650	1600	1340
337	roast (weighed with bone)	1000	1590	1780	550	260	910	750	910	260	1040	1360	520	1230	1880	3370	1040	1000	840
338	**Pigeon** roast	1380	2180	2440	760	360	1240	1020	1240	360	1420	1870	710	1690	2580	4620	1420	1380	1150
339	roast (weighed with bone)	610	960	1070	330	160	550	450	550	160	620	820	310	740	1130	2030	620	610	510
340	**Turkey** raw, meat only	1090	1690	1970	630	250	980	740	910	250	1120	1370	630	1260	2040	3480	1090	1090	910
341	meat and skin	1020	1580	1840	590	230	920	690	860	230	1050	1280	590	1180	1910	3260	1020	1020	860
342	light meat	1150	1780	2080	670	260	1040	780	970	260	1190	1450	670	1340	2150	3670	1150	1150	970
343	dark meat	1000	1560	1810	580	230	910	680	840	230	1040	1260	580	1170	1880	3210	1000	1000	840
344	roast, meat only	1430	2210	2580	830	320	1290	970	1200	320	1480	1800	830	1660	2670	4560	1430	1430	1200
345	meat and skin	1390	2150	2510	810	310	1250	940	1170	310	1430	1750	810	1610	2600	4440	1390	1390	1170
346	light meat	1480	2290	2670	860	330	1330	1000	1240	330	1520	1860	860	1710	2760	4710	1480	1480	1240
347	dark meat	1380	2130	2490	800	310	1240	930	1150	310	1420	1730	800	1600	2580	4400	1380	1380	1150

Other game

No	Food	Ile	Leu	Lys	Met	Cys	Phe	Tyr	Thr	Trp	Val	Arg	His	Ala	Asp	Glu	Gly	Pro	Ser
348	**Hare** stewed	1480	2290	2630	810	380	1390	1100	1290	340	1530	1910	770	1820	2870	4920	1530	1530	1240
349	stewed (weighed with bone)	1080	1670	1910	590	280	1010	800	940	240	1110	1390	560	1320	2090	3580	1110	1110	910
350	**Rabbit** raw	1090	1680	1930	600	280	1020	810	950	250	1120	1400	560	1330	2100	3610	1120	1120	910
351	stewed	1360	2100	2400	740	350	1270	1010	1180	310	1400	1750	700	1660	2620	4500	1400	1400	1140
352	stewed (weighed with bone)	690	1070	1230	380	180	650	510	600	160	710	890	360	850	1340	2300	710	710	580
353	**Venison** roast	1790	2800	3190	950	450	1570	1340	1620	450	1850	2350	1290	2240	3360	6050	1960	1790	1570

23

Meat and meat products *continued*

Amino acids (mg per 100 g food)

No	Food	Ile	Leu	Lys	Met	Cys	Phe	Tyr	Thr	Trp	Val	Arg	His	Ala	Asp	Glu	Gly	Pro	Ser
	Offal																		
354	**Brain, calf and lamb** raw	440	840	920	210	180	530	390	530	130	590	640	410	560	940	1430	480	560	540
355	**calf** boiled	550	1040	1140	260	220	650	490	650	160	730	790	510	690	1160	1770	590	690	670
356	**lamb** boiled	500	950	1040	240	210	600	450	600	150	670	730	470	630	1060	1620	540	630	610
358	**Heart, lamb** raw	900	1560	1470	380	270	790	570	790	220	960	1090	440	1070	1450	2590	1040	600	900
359	**sheep** roast	1380	2380	2260	590	420	1210	880	1210	330	1460	1670	670	1630	2220	3970	1590	920	1380
360	**ox** raw	1000	1730	1640	420	300	880	640	880	240	1060	1210	490	1180	1610	2880	1150	670	1000
361	stewed	1660	2860	2710	700	500	1460	1050	1460	400	1760	2010	800	1960	2660	4770	1910	1100	1660
362	**pig** raw	900	1560	1480	380	270	800	580	800	220	960	1100	440	1070	1450	2600	1040	600	900
364	**Kidney, lamb** raw	690	1290	1350	340	240	820	530	710	210	920	920	580	870	1450	2030	980	920	790
365	fried	1020	1930	2010	510	360	1220	790	1060	320	1380	1380	870	1300	2170	3030	1460	1380	1180
366	**ox** raw	650	1230	1280	330	230	780	500	680	200	880	880	550	830	1380	1930	930	880	750
367	stewed	1060	2000	2090	530	370	1270	820	1100	330	1430	1430	900	1350	2250	3150	1510	1430	1230
368	**pig** raw	680	1280	1330	340	240	810	520	710	210	910	910	570	860	1440	2010	970	910	780
369	stewed	1020	1920	1990	510	350	1210	780	1060	310	1370	1370	860	1290	2150	3010	1450	1370	1170
371	**Liver, calf** raw	870	1570	1700	480	290	1000	610	870	260	1160	1060	740	1060	1730	2440	1000	1060	930
372	fried	1160	2110	2280	650	390	1340	820	1160	350	1550	1420	990	1420	2330	3280	1340	1420	1250
373	**chicken** raw	820	1500	1620	460	280	950	580	820	240	1100	1010	700	1010	1650	2320	950	1010	890
374	fried	890	1620	1750	500	300	1030	630	890	270	1190	1090	760	1090	1790	2520	1030	1090	960
375	**lamb** raw	870	1580	1710	480	290	1000	610	870	260	1160	1060	740	1060	1740	2450	1000	1060	930
376	fried	990	1800	1950	550	330	1140	700	990	290	1320	1210	840	1210	1980	2790	1140	1210	1060
377	**ox** raw	910	1650	1790	510	300	1050	640	910	270	1210	1110	780	1110	1820	2560	1050	1110	980
378	stewed	1070	1940	2100	590	360	1230	750	1070	320	1430	1310	910	1310	2140	3010	1230	1310	1150

Amino acids (mg per 100 g food)

No	Food	Ile	Leu	Lys	Met	Cys	Phe	Tyr	Thr	Trp	Val	Arg	His	Ala	Asp	Glu	Gly	Pro	Ser
	Offal contd																		
379	**Liver, pig** raw	920	1670	1810	510	310	1060	650	920	270	1230	1130	780	1130	1840	2590	1060	1130	990
380	stewed	1100	2000	2170	610	370	1270	780	1100	330	1470	1350	940	1350	2210	3110	1270	1350	1190
381	**Oxtail** raw	960	1380	1790	380	260	800	670	830	260	960	1220	800	1150	1660	3140	1250	1280	800
382	stewed	1460	2100	2730	590	390	1220	1030	1270	390	1460	1850	1220	1760	2540	4780	1900	1950	1220
383	stewed (weighed with bones)	560	800	1040	220	150	460	390	480	150	560	700	460	670	960	1810	720	740	460
384	**Sweetbread, lamb** raw	540	980	1320	220	200	510	370	560	200	660	900	440	780	1050	2120	950	780	610
385	fried	680	1240	1670	280	250	650	470	710	250	780	1150	560	990	1330	2700	1210	990	780
387	**Tongue, lamb** raw	710	1080	1620	270	220	540	470	640	200	740	910	610	810	1320	2400	860	810	640
388	**sheep** stewed	840	1280	1920	320	260	640	550	760	230	870	1080	730	960	1570	2850	1020	960	760
389	**ox** pickled, raw	730	1100	1660	280	230	550	480	650	200	750	930	630	830	1360	2460	880	830	650
390	boiled	910	1370	2060	340	280	690	590	810	250	940	1150	780	1030	1690	3060	1090	1030	810
391	**Tripe** dressed	380	630	750	230	120	360	270	410	120	470	660	270	630	800	1410	980	800	470
392	stewed	590	1000	1190	360	190	570	430	640	190	740	1040	430	1000	1260	2230	1540	1260	740

Meat and meat products *continued*

Amino acids (mg per 100 g food)

No	Food	Ile	Leu	Lys	Met	Cys	Phe	Tyr	Thr	Trp	Val	Arg	His	Ala	Asp	Glu	Gly	Pro	Ser
	Meat products and dishes																		
	Canned meats																		
393	**Beef, corned**	1250	1980	2490	650	390	1120	1030	1200	390	1420	1760	770	1680	2490	4390	1810	1680	1080
394	**Ham**	860	1420	1650	500	240	740	590	800	180	920	1210	680	1120	1680	3040	1150	940	680
395	**Ham and pork** chopped	620	990	1220	320	180	530	480	620	160	690	940	460	850	1310	2300	1010	920	640
396	**Luncheon meat**	470	790	830	240	180	490	340	440	160	590	770	300	790	970	1940	1090	1110	550
397	**Stewed steak with gravy**	640	1040	1280	330	170	590	430	660	170	690	950	500	880	1260	2490	1020	920	690
398	**Tongue**	740	1180	1540	380	230	770	590	690	230	820	1050	380	970	1380	2460	1100	1000	720
400	**Veal, jellied**	1200	1800	2160	600	320	1080	840	1080	280	1240	1720	720	1440	2200	3960	1560	1360	1080
	Offal products																		
401	**Black pudding** fried	290	1260	950	190	170	740	310	520	170	930	620	640	950	1220	1920	820	910	620
402	**Faggots**	450	780	750	180	160	530	250	390	130	570	710	250	800	850	2260	1100	1140	520
403	**Haggis** boiled	410	790	720	170	140	460	290	450	120	630	650	290	630	870	1730	750	720	510
404	**Liver sausage**	520	970	1010	250	170	560	350	700	140	760	760	430	760	1070	2020	1010	780	640
	Sausages																		
405	**Frankfurters**	440	700	750	210	110	410	320	380	91	490	620	270	610	850	1630	730	750	430
406	**Polony**	360	620	690	180	110	350	210	330	110	450	540	230	530	690	2010	740	830	380
407	**Salami**	930	1390	1610	400	250	800	590	870	220	960	1170	530	1140	1790	3280	1330	1140	770
408	**Sausages, beef** raw	400	660	590	190	150	400	250	370	120	480	590	250	620	770	1970	850	850	420
409	fried	540	890	790	250	210	540	330	500	170	640	790	330	830	1040	2650	1140	1140	560
410	grilled	540	890	790	250	210	540	330	500	170	650	790	330	830	1040	2660	1140	1140	560
411	**Sausages, pork** raw	440	690	690	220	190	420	270	410	140	510	630	290	630	830	1940	780	860	460
412	fried	570	900	900	290	240	550	350	530	180	660	810	370	810	1080	2530	1010	1120	590
413	grilled	550	870	870	280	230	530	340	510	170	640	790	360	790	1040	2450	980	1090	580
414	**Saveloy**	350	600	730	180	130	330	240	330	110	430	590	250	570	750	1590	840	810	380

Meat and meat products *continued*

Amino acids (mg per 100 g food)

No	Food	Ile	Leu	Lys	Met	Cys	Phe	Tyr	Thr	Trp	Val	Arg	His	Ala	Asp	Glu	Gly	Pro	Ser
	Meat products and dishes contd																		
415	**Beefburgers** frozen, raw	680	1090	1190	390	170	660	490	610	170	750	970	490	970	1310	2840	1020	970	630
416	fried	920	1470	1600	520	230	830	650	820	230	1010	1310	650	1310	1770	3830	1370	1310	850
417	**Brawn**	400	680	900	220	140	540	320	380	140	520	880	260	900	920	1790	1550	880	500
418	**Meat paste**	730	1090	1190	370	190	580	340	970	170	800	950	410	1000	1410	2550	1050	1000	660
419	**White pudding**	280	500	350	130	100	330	210	340	78	430	440	210	330	550	1490	410	450	380
	Meat and pastry products																		
420	**Cornish pastie**	290	510	320	140	130	370	220	260	100	360	330	180	320	510	2150	360	730	320
421	**Pork pie** individual	410	620	520	190	160	480	270	330	130	440	520	250	500	670	2170	610	890	440
422	**Sausage roll** flaky pastry	300	520	310	140	170	340	190	250	90	340	350	180	330	450	1970	390	800	380
423	short pastry	340	580	340	160	190	380	220	280	100	390	390	200	370	500	2240	430	900	430
424	**Steak and kidney pie** pastry top only	730	1210	1220	370	230	720	540	660	190	810	930	530	870	1340	2830	820	970	730
425	individual	420	750	500	180	160	560	190	370	100	530	560	280	530	660	2470	570	1040	420
	Cooked dishes																		
426	**Beef steak pudding**	530	860	840	270	170	500	400	470	140	560	680	370	620	930	2270	560	730	520
427	**Beef stew**	490	760	850	260	130	430	370	440	120	500	650	350	600	900	1720	530	510	430
428	**Bolognese sauce**	380	590	670	200	96	330	280	350	97	400	500	270	470	760	1260	410	380	340
429	**Curried meat**	530	850	850	280	160	500	400	470	140	560	700	370	630	950	2210	560	690	510
430	**Hot pot**	460	710	800	240	120	410	350	420	120	480	620	320	550	950	1570	490	450	400
431	**Irish stew**	230	360	460	120	64	200	180	230	68	250	320	150	270	540	830	230	230	220
432	**Irish stew** (weighed with bones)	210	330	420	110	58	190	170	210	63	230	300	140	250	500	770	210	210	200
433	**Moussaka**	470	760	770	240	110	430	360	420	130	530	550	300	500	900	1690	410	560	450
434	**Shepherd's pie**	390	610	680	200	98	350	290	350	100	410	510	270	470	790	1320	410	390	340

Fish and fish products

Amino acids (mg per 100 g food)

No	Food	Ile	Leu	Lys	Met	Cys	Phe	Tyr	Thr	Trp	Val	Arg	His	Ala	Asp	Glu	Gly	Pro	Ser
	White fish																		
438	**Cod** raw, fresh fillets	920	1470	1700	500	200	720	610	830	200	1000	1110	500	1200	1810	2640	810	720	860
439	frozen steaks	820	1320	1520	450	170	650	550	750	170	900	1000	450	1070	1620	2370	720	650	770
440	baked	1130	1820	2090	620	240	890	760	1030	240	1240	1370	620	1480	2230	3260	1000	890	1060
441	baked (weighed with bones and skin)	960	1550	1780	530	200	760	640	880	200	1050	1170	530	1260	1900	2770	850	760	910
442	fried in batter	1040	1660	1920	570	220	820	690	940	220	1130	1260	570	1350	2040	2980	910	820	970
443	grilled	1100	1760	2030	600	230	860	730	1000	230	1200	1330	600	1430	2160	3150	960	860	1030
444	poached	1110	1780	2040	600	240	870	740	1010	240	1210	1340	600	1440	2180	3180	970	870	1040
445	poached (weighed with bones and skin)	960	1540	1780	520	200	760	640	870	200	1050	1160	520	1250	1890	2770	840	760	900
446	steamed	980	1580	1820	540	210	780	660	890	210	1070	1190	540	1280	1940	2830	860	780	920
447	steamed (weighed with bones and skin)	800	1280	1480	440	170	630	530	730	170	870	970	440	1040	1570	2300	700	630	750
448	**smoked** raw	970	1550	1790	530	210	760	650	880	210	1060	1170	530	1260	1910	2780	850	760	910
449	poached	1140	1830	2110	620	240	900	760	1040	240	1250	1380	620	1490	2250	3290	1000	900	1070
450	**dried** salt, boiled	1720	2760	3170	940	360	1350	1140	1560	360	1870	2080	940	2240	3380	4940	1510	1350	1610
451	**Haddock, fresh** raw	880	1420	1640	480	190	700	590	800	190	970	1070	480	1150	1740	2550	780	700	830
452	fried	1130	1810	2090	620	240	890	750	1030	240	1230	1370	620	1470	2220	3250	990	890	1060
453	fried (weighed with bones)	1040	1670	1920	570	220	820	690	950	220	1130	1260	570	1360	2050	2990	910	820	980
454	steamed	1210	1940	2230	660	260	950	800	1100	260	1310	1460	660	1570	2370	3470	1060	950	1130
455	steamed (weighed with bones and skin)	910	1470	1690	500	190	720	610	830	190	1000	1110	500	1190	1800	2630	800	720	860
456	**smoked** steamed	1230	1980	2280	670	260	970	820	1120	260	1340	1490	670	1600	2430	3540	1080	970	1160
457	steamed (weighed with bones and skin)	800	1280	1480	440	170	630	530	730	170	870	970	440	1040	1570	2300	700	630	750

Fish and fish products *continued*

Amino acids (mg per 100 g food)

No	Food	Ile	Leu	Lys	Met	Cys	Phe	Tyr	Thr	Trp	Val	Arg	His	Ala	Asp	Glu	Gly	Pro	Ser
	White fish contd																		
458	**Halibut** raw	930	1500	1730	510	200	740	620	850	200	1020	1130	510	1220	1840	2690	820	740	880
459	steamed	1250	2010	2320	680	270	990	840	1140	270	1370	1520	680	1630	2470	3610	1100	990	1180
460	steamed (weighed with bones and skin)	950	1530	1760	520	200	750	630	860	200	1040	1150	520	1240	1870	2740	840	750	890
461	**Lemon sole** raw	900	1450	1670	490	190	710	600	820	190	990	1100	490	1180	1780	2600	800	710	850
462	fried	850	1360	1570	460	180	670	570	770	180	930	1030	460	1110	1670	2440	750	670	800
463	fried (weighed with bones)	670	1080	1240	370	140	530	450	610	140	730	810	370	870	1320	1930	590	530	630
464	steamed	1090	1740	2010	590	230	860	720	990	230	1180	1320	590	1420	2140	3130	950	860	1020
465	steamed (weighed with bones and skin)	770	1240	1430	420	160	610	520	700	160	840	940	420	1010	1520	2220	680	610	730
466	**Plaice** raw	940	1520	1750	520	200	740	630	860	200	1030	1140	520	1230	1860	2720	830	740	890
467	fried in batter	830	1340	1540	450	180	660	550	760	180	910	1010	450	1080	1640	2390	730	660	780
468	fried in crumbs	950	1530	1760	520	200	750	630	860	200	1040	1150	520	1240	1870	2740	840	750	890
469	steamed	1000	1600	1840	540	210	790	660	910	210	1090	1210	540	1300	1960	2870	880	790	940
470	steamed (weighed with bones and skin)	540	860	990	290	110	420	360	490	110	590	650	290	700	1060	1550	470	420	510
471	**Saithe** raw	900	1440	1660	490	190	710	600	820	190	980	1090	490	1170	1770	2580	790	710	840
472	steamed	1230	1980	2280	670	260	970	820	1120	260	1340	1490	670	1600	2430	3540	1080	970	1160
473	steamed (weighed with bones and skin)	1050	1680	1930	570	220	820	700	950	220	1140	1270	570	1360	2060	3010	920	820	980
475	**Whiting** fried	960	1540	1770	520	200	750	640	870	200	1040	1160	520	1250	1890	2760	840	750	900
476	fried (weighed with bones)	860	1380	1590	470	180	680	570	780	180	940	1040	470	1120	1700	2480	760	680	810
477	steamed	1110	1780	2040	600	240	870	740	1010	240	1210	1340	600	1440	2180	3180	970	870	1040
478	steamed (weighed with bones)	750	1210	1390	410	160	590	500	680	160	820	910	410	980	1430	2170	660	590	710

Fish and fish products *continued*

Amino acids (mg per 100 g food)

No	Food	Ile	Leu	Lys	Met	Cys	Phe	Tyr	Thr	Trp	Val	Arg	His	Ala	Asp	Glu	Gly	Pro	Ser
	Fatty fish																		
480	**Eel** raw	880	1410	1620	480	190	690	590	800	190	960	1060	480	1140	1730	2530	770	690	830
481	stewed	1090	1750	2010	590	230	860	730	990	230	1190	1320	590	1420	2150	3140	960	860	1020
482	**Herring** raw	890	1430	1640	480	190	700	590	810	190	970	1080	480	1160	1750	2560	780	700	830
483	fried	1220	1960	2250	660	260	960	810	1110	260	1330	1480	660	1590	2400	3510	1070	960	1140
484	fried (weighed with bones)	1070	1720	1980	580	230	840	710	970	230	1170	1300	580	1390	2110	3080	940	840	1000
485	grilled	1080	1730	1990	590	230	850	720	980	230	1170	1300	590	1400	2120	3100	950	850	1010
486	grilled (weighed with bones)	730	1180	1350	400	160	580	490	670	160	800	890	400	960	1440	2110	640	580	690
487	**Bloater** grilled	1240	1990	2290	680	260	980	830	1130	260	1350	1500	680	1620	2440	3570	1090	980	1170
488	grilled (weighed with bones)	920	1470	1700	500	200	720	610	830	200	1000	1110	500	1200	1810	2640	810	720	860
489	**Kipper** baked	1350	2160	2490	730	290	1060	900	1220	290	1470	1630	730	1750	2650	3880	1180	1060	1270
490	baked (weighed with bones)	730	1170	1340	400	150	570	480	660	150	790	880	400	950	1430	2090	640	570	680
491	**Mackerel** raw	1000	1610	1850	550	210	790	670	910	210	1090	1220	550	1310	1980	2890	880	790	940
492	fried	1140	1820	2100	620	240	890	760	1030	240	1240	1380	620	1480	2240	3270	1000	890	1070
493	fried (weighed with bones)	830	1330	1530	450	180	650	550	750	180	900	1000	450	1080	1630	2390	730	650	780
494	**Pilchards** canned in tomato sauce	990	1600	1840	540	210	780	660	900	210	1080	1200	540	1290	1960	2860	870	780	930
495	**Salmon** raw	970	1560	1790	530	210	760	650	880	210	1060	1180	530	1260	1910	2790	850	760	910
496	steamed	1060	1700	1960	580	230	840	710	960	230	1160	1280	580	1380	2090	3050	930	840	1000
497	steamed (weighed with bones and skin)	860	1380	1590	470	180	680	570	780	180	940	1040	470	1120	1690	2470	750	680	810

Fish and fish products *continued*

No	Food	Ile	Leu	Lys	Met	Cys	Phe	Tyr	Thr	Trp	Val	Arg	His	Ala	Asp	Glu	Gly	Pro	Ser
	Fatty fish conta																		
498	**Salmon** canned	1070	1720	1980	580	230	840	710	970	230	1170	1300	580	1390	2110	3080	940	840	1000
499	smoked	1340	2150	2480	730	280	1060	890	1220	280	1460	1620	730	1750	2640	3860	1180	1060	1260
500	**Sardines** canned in oil, fish only	1250	2010	2310	680	270	990	830	1140	270	1360	1520	680	1630	2460	3600	1100	990	1180
501	fish plus oil	1040	1670	1920	570	220	820	690	950	220	1130	1260	570	1360	2050	2990	910	820	980
502	canned in tomato sauce	940	1510	1730	510	200	740	630	850	200	1020	1140	510	1220	1850	2700	820	740	880
504	**Sprats** fried	1310	2110	2430	720	280	1040	880	1190	280	1430	1590	720	1710	2590	3780	1150	1040	1230
505	fried (weighed with bones)	1160	1860	2140	630	250	910	770	1050	250	1260	1400	630	1510	2280	3330	1020	910	1090
506	**Trout, brown** steamed	1240	1990	2290	680	260	980	830	1130	260	1350	1500	680	1620	2440	3570	1090	980	1170
507	steamed (weighed with bones)	820	1310	1510	450	170	650	550	740	170	890	990	450	1070	1610	2360	720	650	770
508	**Tuna** canned in oil	1210	1940	2230	660	260	950	800	1100	260	1310	1460	660	1570	2370	3470	1060	950	1130
509	**Whitebait** fried	1030	1650	1900	560	220	810	690	940	220	1120	1250	560	1340	2030	2960	910	810	970
	Cartilaginous fish																		
511	**Dogfish** fried in batter	1130	1810	2090	620	240	890	750	1030	240	1230	1370	620	1470	2220	3250	990	890	1060
512	fried (weighed with waste)	1040	1670	1920	570	220	820	690	950	220	1130	1260	570	1360	2050	2990	910	820	980
514	**Skate** fried in batter	1210	1950	2240	660	260	950	810	1100	260	1320	1470	660	1580	2390	3490	1060	950	1140
515	fried (weighed with waste)	990	1600	1840	540	210	780	660	900	210	1080	1200	540	1290	1960	2860	870	780	930

Fish and fish products *continued*

Amino acids (mg per 100 g food)

No	Food	Ile	Leu	Lys	Met	Cys	Phe	Tyr	Thr	Trp	Val	Arg	His	Ala	Asp	Glu	Gly	Pro	Ser
	Crustacea																		
518	**Crab** boiled	930	1730	1570	580	260	800	740	930	230	960	1670	390	1350	2180	3150	1320	870	1030
519	boiled (weighed with shell)	190	350	310	120	51	160	150	190	45	190	330	77	270	440	630	260	170	210
520	canned	840	1570	1420	520	230	730	670	840	200	870	1510	350	1220	1970	2840	1190	780	930
521	**Lobster** boiled	1030	1910	1740	640	280	890	810	1030	250	1060	1840	430	1490	2410	3470	1450	960	1130
522	boiled (weighed with shell)	370	690	620	230	100	320	290	370	89	380	660	150	530	860	1250	520	340	410
523	**Prawns** boiled	1050	1960	1770	650	290	910	830	1050	250	1090	1880	430	1520	2460	3550	1480	980	1160
524	boiled (weighed with shell)	400	750	680	250	110	350	320	400	97	410	720	170	580	940	1350	570	370	440
525	**Scampi** fried	570	1050	960	350	160	490	450	570	140	590	1010	230	820	1330	1910	800	530	620
527	**Shrimps** boiled	1100	2050	1860	680	300	950	870	1100	270	1140	1980	460	1600	2580	3720	1560	1030	1220
528	boiled (weighed with shell)	370	680	620	230	100	320	290	370	88	380	660	150	530	860	1240	520	340	400
529	canned	970	1800	1630	600	270	830	770	970	230	1000	1730	400	1400	2260	3260	1370	900	1070
	Molluscs																		
531	**Cockles** boiled	540	860	900	310	180	470	470	520	140	700	850	270	630	1260	1580	580	470	580
532	**Mussels** raw	580	930	970	330	190	500	500	560	150	750	910	290	680	1350	1700	620	500	620
533	boiled	830	1320	1380	470	280	720	720	800	220	1070	1290	410	960	1930	2420	880	720	880
534	boiled (weighed with shell)	250	400	420	140	83	220	220	240	66	320	390	130	290	580	730	270	220	270
535	**Oysters** raw	520	830	860	290	170	450	450	500	140	670	810	260	600	1200	1510	550	450	550
536	raw (weighed with shell)	63	100	110	36	21	55	55	61	17	82	99	32	74	150	190	67	55	67
538	**Scallops** steamed	1110	1780	1860	630	370	970	970	1080	300	1450	1740	560	1300	2600	3270	1190	970	1190

Fish and fish products *continued*

No	Fcod	Ile	Leu	Lys	Met	Cys	Phe	Tyr	Thr	Trp	Val	Arg	His	Ala	Asp	Glu	Gly	Pro	Ser
	Molluscs contd																		
539	**Whelks** boiled	890	1420	1480	500	300	770	770	860	240	1150	1390	440	1040	2070	2610	950	770	950
540	boiled (weighed with shell)	130	210	220	75	44	110	110	130	35	170	210	66	150	310	390	140	110	140
541	**Winkles** boiled	740	1180	1230	420	250	640	640	710	200	960	1150	370	860	1720	2160	780	640	780
542	boiled (weighed with shell)	140	230	240	80	47	120	120	140	38	180	220	71	170	330	410	150	120	150
	Fish products and dishes																		
545	**Fish fingers** frozen	600	1000	850	300	210	560	400	510	140	660	670	330	680	1020	2790	520	940	660
546	fried	670	1100	1070	350	200	580	450	580	150	730	770	360	810	1210	2610	580	830	690
548	**Fish pie**	360	590	630	190	82	310	250	330	84	410	420	200	430	780	1140	300	340	350
549	**Kedgeree**	680	1070	1130	370	160	560	460	610	60	780	810	350	830	1330	1860	550	520	700

Amino acids (mg per 100 g food)

No	Food	Ile	Leu	Lys	Met	Cys	Phe	Tyr	Thr	Trp	Val	Arg	His	Ala	Asp	Glu	Gly	Pro	Ser
558	**Asparagus** boiled	86	150	150	43	32	86	70	97	38	120	130	54	190	370	700	110	190	110
559	boiled (weighed as served)	43	76	76	22	16	43	35	49	19	62	65	27	97	180	350	57	97	54
561	**Beans, French** boiled	28	52	41	10	8	32	25	29	11	37	32	18	34	90	80	29	29	40
562	**runner** raw	83	160	120	29	25	97	76	86	32	110	97	54	100	270	240	86	86	120
563	boiled	71	130	110	25	22	84	65	74	28	96	84	47	87	230	210	74	74	100
564	**broad** boiled	170	290	260	26	33	180	130	140	40	190	370	99	170	460	620	170	170	190
565	**butter** raw	950	1560	1440	280	280	1160	610	800	180	980	1130	610	890	2360	2510	800	890	1260
566	boiled	350	580	530	100	100	430	230	290	68	360	420	230	330	870	930	290	330	460
567	**haricot** raw	890	1640	1540	240	170	1130	550	860	210	990	1230	620	890	2570	3150	820	750	1200
568	boiled	280	510	480	74	53	350	170	270	64	310	380	190	280	800	980	250	230	370
569	**baked** canned in tomato sauce	210	390	370	57	41	270	130	210	49	240	300	150	210	620	750	200	180	290

Vegetables *continued*

Amino acids (mg per 100 g food)

No	Food	Ile	Leu	Lys	Met	Cys	Phe	Tyr	Thr	Trp	Val	Arg	His	Ala	Asp	Glu	Gly	Pro	Ser
572	**Beans, red kidney** raw	920	1700	1590	250	180	1170	570	890	210	1030	1270	640	920	2660	3260	850	780	1240
574	**Beetroot** raw	32	59	69	25	15	46	46	44	13	32	86	17	29	240	200	27	34	46
575	boiled	44	81	96	35	20	64	64	61	17	44	120	23	41	330	280	38	46	64
576	**Broccoli tops** raw	130	170	170	47	36	120	N	120	36	160	190	57	N	N	N	N	N	N
577	boiled	120	160	160	44	34	110	N	110	34	150	180	54	N	N	N	N	N	N
578	**Brussels sprouts** raw	170	220	220	38	26	150	N	170	45	190	250	90	N	N	N	N	N	N
579	boiled	120	150	150	27	18	100	N	120	32	140	180	63	N	N	N	N	N	N
580	**Cabbage, red** raw	51	89	51	16	19	51	32	62	16	70	140	43	86	110	150	81	62	70
581	**Savoy,** raw	100	180	100	32	37	100	64	120	32	140	280	85	170	220	290	160	120	140
582	boiled	40	69	40	13	15	40	25	48	13	55	110	34	67	86	110	63	48	55
583	**spring** boiled	34	59	34	11	13	34	22	41	11	47	94	29	58	74	97	54	41	47
584	**white** raw	59	100	59	19	22	59	37	71	19	81	160	50	99	130	170	93	71	81
585	**winter** raw	86	150	86	27	32	86	54	100	27	120	230	72	140	190	240	140	100	120
586	boiled	51	89	51	16	19	51	32	62	16	70	140	43	86	110	150	81	62	70

Vegetables *continued*

No	Food	Ile	Leu	Lys	Met	Cys	Phe	Tyr	Thr	Trp	Val	Arg	His	Ala	Asp	Glu	Gly	Pro	Ser
587	**Carrots, old** raw	21	31	26	8	8	19	15	20	6	31	31	10	33	80	130	20	20	22
588	boiled	19	28	24	7	7	17	14	18	5	28	28	9	30	73	120	18	18	20
589	**young** boiled	27	39	34	10	10	24	20	25	7	39	39	13	42	100	170	25	25	28
590	canned	21	31	26	8	8	19	15	20	6	31	31	10	33	80	130	20	20	22
591	**Cauliflower** raw	81	130	110	36	N	63	27	78	27	110	84	36	150	160	140	130	N	N
592	boiled	70	110	91	31	N	55	23	68	23	94	73	31	130	140	130	110	N	N
594	**Celery** raw	36	65	20	17	5	42	12	32	11	45	38	14	N	N	N	N	N	N
595	boiled	24	43	13	11	3	28	8	21	7	30	25	9	N	N	N	N	N	N
597	**Cucumber** raw	19	26	27	6	N	14	N	16	5	21	47	9	N	N	N	N	N	N
603	**Lentils** raw	1030	1820	1710	190	230	1250	760	950	230	1180	2050	650	1030	2740	3950	990	1030	1250
604	split, boiled	330	590	550	61	73	400	240	310	73	380	660	210	330	880	1270	320	330	400
605	masur dahl, cooked	210	370	350	39	47	260	160	200	47	240	420	130	210	560	810	200	210	260

Vegetables *continued*

No	Food	Ile	Leu	Lys	Met	Cys	Phe	Tyr	Thr	Trp	Val	Arg	His	Ala	Asp	Glu	Gly	Pro	Ser
606	**Lettuce** raw	38	62	38	18	N	51	27	42	8	54	45	16	43	120	100	42	53	34
609	**Mushrooms** raw	90	150	180	58	32	83	77	110	38	100	240	51	190	180	280	100	210	110
610	fried	130	210	250	81	45	120	110	150	54	140	330	72	260	250	400	140	290	150
613	**Onions** raw	14	26	42	11	N	26	32	14	14	21	120	9	N	N	140	N	N	N
614	boiled	8	15	25	6	N	15	19	8	8	13	72	5	N	N	84	N	N	N
615	fried	26	49	81	20	N	49	61	26	26	41	230	17	N	N	270	N	N	N
616	spring, raw	14	26	42	11	N	26	32	14	14	21	120	9	N	N	140	N	N	N
620	**Peas, fresh** raw	250	400	430	55	64	270	160	230	55	270	540	130	240	640	930	230	220	250
621	boiled	220	340	380	48	56	230	140	200	48	230	470	110	210	550	810	200	190	220
622	**frozen** raw	250	390	430	55	64	260	160	230	55	260	540	130	240	630	920	230	220	250
623	boiled	240	370	410	52	61	250	150	220	52	250	510	120	230	600	880	220	210	240
624	**canned** garden	200	320	350	44	52	220	130	190	44	220	440	100	190	510	750	190	180	200
625	processed	270	430	470	59	69	290	170	250	59	290	580	140	260	680	1000	250	240	270

Vegetables *continued*

Amino acids (mg per 100 g food)

No	Food	Ile	Leu	Lys	Met	Cys	Phe	Tyr	Thr	Trp	Val	Arg	His	Ala	Asp	Glu	Gly	Pro	Ser
626	**Peas, dried** raw	930	1480	1620	210	240	1000	590	860	210	1000	2040	480	900	2380	3490	860	830	930
627	boiled	300	480	520	67	78	320	190	280	67	320	660	160	290	770	1120	280	270	300
628	**split** dried, raw	960	1520	1660	210	250	1030	600	890	210	1030	2090	500	920	2440	3580	890	850	960
629	boiled	360	570	630	80	93	390	230	330	80	390	790	190	350	920	1340	330	320	360
630	**chick** Bengal gram, raw	900	1520	1390	260	290	1160	580	780	160	900	1910	550	870	2360	3200	810	840	1030
631	cooked, dahl	360	600	550	100	120	460	230	310	64	360	760	220	350	930	1270	320	330	410
632	channa dahl	240	400	370	68	77	310	150	200	43	240	500	150	230	620	840	210	220	270
633	**red** pigeon, raw	610	1250	1540	260	220	1660	420	580	96	740	960	740	830	1920	3740	640	800	830
639	**Potatoes, old** raw	88	130	120	34	27	92	65	82	31	110	110	41	78	390	270	71	82	88
640	boiled	60	87	78	23	18	62	44	55	21	74	71	28	53	270	180	48	55	60
641	mashed	62	91	82	24	19	65	46	58	22	77	74	29	55	280	190	50	58	62
642	baked	110	160	140	41	33	110	78	98	37	130	130	49	94	470	330	86	98	110
643	baked (weighed with skins)	86	130	110	33	26	89	63	79	30	110	100	40	76	380	260	69	79	86
644	roast	120	170	150	45	36	120	86	110	41	140	140	54	100	520	360	95	110	120
645	chips	160	230	210	61	49	170	120	150	55	200	190	73	140	700	490	130	150	160

Vegetables *continued*

No	Food	Ile	Leu	Lys	Met	Cys	Phe	Tyr	Thr	Trp	Val	Arg	His	Ala	Asp	Glu	Gly	Pro	Ser
646	**Potatoes, old** chips, frozen	91	130	120	35	28	95	67	84	32	110	110	42	81	400	280	74	84	91
647	frozen, fried	130	180	160	48	38	130	91	120	43	150	150	58	110	550	380	100	120	130
648	**new** boiled	65	95	85	25	20	68	48	60	23	80	78	30	58	290	200	53	60	65
649	canned	49	72	65	19	15	51	36	46	17	61	59	23	44	220	150	40	46	49
650	**instant** powder	380	550	490	150	120	390	280	350	130	460	450	170	330	1670	1160	310	350	380
651	made up	83	120	110	32	26	86	61	77	29	100	99	38	74	370	260	67	77	83
652	**crisps**	260	380	340	100	80	270	190	240	90	320	310	120	230	1150	800	210	240	260
657	**Spinach** boiled	240	480	370	89	81	310	250	270	81	310	320	130	320	500	590	260	240	240
658	**Spring greens** boiled	43	70	32	19	12	35	24	49	22	43	27	14	73	97	160	43	59	57
661	**Sweetcorn, on the cob** raw	150	520	110	79	66	210	160	150	26	200	170	110	310	260	780	150	370	210
662	boiled	150	510	110	78	65	200	160	150	26	200	170	110	310	250	770	150	360	200
663	**canned** kernels	110	370	80	56	47	150	110	110	19	140	120	80	220	180	560	110	260	150

Vegetables *continued*

Amino acids (mg per 100 g food)

No	Food	Ile	Leu	Lys	Met	Cys	Phe	Tyr	Thr	Trp	Val	Arg	His	Ala	Asp	Glu	Gly	Pro	Ser
664	**Sweet potatoes** raw	44	65	40	19	13	46	29	46	21	53	59	15	57	160	100	44	42	49
665	boiled	39	58	36	17	12	41	26	41	19	48	53	14	51	140	92	39	37	44
666	**Tomatoes** raw	17	24	25	6	6	15	11	20	7	18	18	13	21	100	N	15	14	22
667	fried	19	27	29	6	6	18	13	22	8	21	21	14	24	120	N	18	16	26
668	canned	20	29	31	7	7	19	14	24	9	22	22	15	26	120	N	19	17	27
669	**Turnips** raw	19	31	14	8	N	16	11	22	10	19	12	6	35	43	70	19	26	25
670	boiled	18	29	13	8	N	14	10	20	9	18	11	6	32	40	64	18	24	23
671	**Turnip tops** boiled	90	180	130	39	34	120	73	110	34	120	100	47	140	210	290	120	110	99
673	**Yam** raw	70	120	83	29	26	93	64	67	26	86	150	38	86	210	250	70	74	100
674	boiled	55	95	65	23	20	73	50	53	20	68	120	30	68	170	200	55	58	80

Fruit Amino acids (mg per 100 g food)

No	Food	Ile	Leu	Lys	Met	Cys	Phe	Tyr	Thr	Trp	Val	Arg	His	Ala	Asp	Glu	Gly	Pro	Ser
675	**Apples, eating**																		
676	eating (weighed with skin and core)	9	16	15	2	3	6	4	9	2	10	7	5	11	52	28	10	8	11
677	**cooking** raw	7	12	11	2	2	5	3	7	2	8	5	4	8	39	21	7	6	8
678	baked without sugar	11	20	19	3	4	8	5	12	3	13	9	6	14	65	35	12	10	14
679	baked (weighed with skin)	11	20	19	3	4	8	5	12	3	13	9	6	14	65	35	12	10	14
680	stewed without sugar	9	16	15	2	3	6	5	9	2	10	7	5	11	52	28	10	8	11
681	stewed with sugar	9	16	15	2	3	6	4	9	2	10	7	5	11	52	28	10	8	11
682	**Apricots** fresh, raw	10	16	16	3	N	9	7	12	5	14	7	9	20	130	33	10	15	16
683	raw (weighed with stones)	9	14	14	2	N	8	6	10	4	12	6	8	18	120	30	9	14	14
684	stewed without sugar	8	13	13	2	N	7	6	9	4	11	6	7	15	100	26	8	12	13
685	stewed without sugar (weighed with stones)	8	13	13	2	N	7	6	9	4	11	6	7	15	100	26	8	12	13
686	stewed with sugar	7	11	11	2	N	6	5	8	3	9	5	6	13	88	22	7	10	11
687	stewed with sugar (weighed with stones)	7	11	11	2	N	6	5	8	3	9	5	6	13	88	22	7	10	11

Fruit *continued*

Amino acids (mg per 100 g food)

No	Food	Ile	Leu	Lys	Met	Cys	Phe	Tyr	Thr	Trp	Val	Arg	His	Ala	Asp	Glu	Gly	Pro	Ser
688	**Apricots** dried, raw	84	140	140	23	N	76	61	99	38	110	61	76	170	1120	280	84	130	140
689	stewed without sugar	31	50	50	8	N	28	22	36	14	42	22	28	62	410	100	31	48	50
690	stewed with sugar	30	49	49	8	N	27	22	35	14	41	22	27	59	400	100	30	46	49
691	canned	9	14	14	2	N	8	6	10	4	12	6	8	18	120	30	9	14	14
692	**Avocado pears**	140	230	210	67	N	150	94	120	47	190	140	74	260	950	520	170	160	170
693	**Bananas** raw	45	58	49	14	31	47	29	34	13	47	65	68	50	120	100	47	47	43
694	raw (weighed with skins)	28	35	30	9	19	29	18	21	8	29	40	42	31	73	64	29	29	26
717	**Currants** dried	14	35	38	57	27	35	30	46	8	46	120	62	70	210	350	51	57	31
724	**Dates** dried	45	86	54	26	42	58	29	54	54	64	67	29	93	120	210	90	120	57
725	dried (weighed with stones)	39	76	48	22	36	50	25	48	48	56	59	25	81	100	180	78	100	59
726	**Figs, green** raw	40	57	53	11	21	32	57	42	11	50	29	19	80	320	130	44	86	65
727	**dried** raw	110	150	140	29	57	86	150	110	29	140	80	51	220	860	340	120	230	180
728	stewed without sugar	61	86	80	16	32	48	86	64	16	77	45	29	120	480	190	67	130	99
729	stewed with sugar	57	81	75	15	30	45	81	60	15	72	42	27	110	450	180	73	120	93
736	**Grapes, black** raw	5	12	13	19	9	12	10	15	3	15	41	21	23	68	120	17	19	27
737	raw (whole grapes weighed)	4	10	11	17	8	10	9	14	2	14	37	18	21	61	100	15	17	24

Fruit *continued*

Amino acids (mg per 100 g food)

No	Food	Ile	Leu	Lys	Met	Cys	Phe	Tyr	Thr	Trp	Val	Arg	His	Ala	Asp	Glu	Gly	Pro	Ser
738	**Grapes, white** raw	5	13	14	21	10	13	11	17	3	17	46	23	26	76	130	19	21	30
739	raw (whole grapes weighed)	5	13	14	21	10	13	11	17	3	17	46	23	26	76	130	19	21	30
740	**Grapefruit** raw	18	17	33	9	8	23	13	9	4	24	40	9	39	88	76	64	35	18
741	raw (whole fruit weighed)	9	9	17	5	4	12	7	5	2	12	20	5	20	44	38	32	18	9
742	canned	14	14	26	7	6	18	10	7	3	19	32	7	31	70	61	51	28	14
749	**Guavas** canned	11	10	20	5	5	14	8	5	2	14	24	5	23	53	46	38	21	11
750	**Lemons** whole	22	20	40	11	10	28	16	11	5	29	48	11	47	110	91	77	42	22
758	**Mandarin oranges** canned	18	17	33	9	8	23	13	9	4	24	40	9	39	88	76	64	35	18
762	**Melons, Cantelloupe** raw	N	N	26	3	N	30	N	N	2	N	N	N	N	N	N	N	N	N
763	raw (weighed with skin)	N	N	16	2	N	19	N	N	1	N	N	N	N	N	N	N	N	N
764	**yellow, Honeydew** raw	N	N	16	2	N	19	N	N	1	N	N	N	N	N	N	N	N	N
765	raw (weighed with skin)	N	N	10	1	N	11	N	N	1	N	N	N	N	N	N	N	N	N
766	**watermelon** raw	N	N	N	N	N	9	9	N	N	N	N	N	N	N	N	N	N	N
769	**Nectarines** raw	15	33	35	36	11	21	24	32	5	47	20	20	47	110	170	18	32	39
770	raw (weighed with stones)	14	31	32	34	10	20	22	29	4	43	18	18	43	99	150	17	29	36

No	Food	Ile	Leu	Lys	Met	Cys	Phe	Tyr	Thr	Trp	Val	Arg	His	Ala	Asp	Glu	Gly	Pro	Ser
773	**Oranges** raw	23	22	43	12	10	30	17	12	5	31	52	12	51	110	99	83	46	23
774	raw (weighed with peel and pips)	18	17	33	9	8	23	13	9	4	24	40	9	39	88	76	64	35	18
775	juice, fresh	18	17	33	9	8	23	13	9	4	24	40	9	39	88	76	64	35	18
779	**Peaches** fresh raw	10	22	23	24	7	14	16	21	3	31	13	13	31	71	110	12	21	26
780	raw (weighed with stones)	9	20	21	22	6	13	14	19	3	28	12	12	28	64	99	11	19	23
781	dried, raw	55	120	130	130	39	77	88	120	17	170	72	72	170	390	610	66	120	140
782	stewed without sugar	20	44	46	48	14	28	32	42	6	62	26	26	62	140	220	24	42	52
783	stewed with sugar	20	44	46	48	14	28	32	42	6	62	26	26	62	140	220	24	42	52
784	canned	6	13	14	14	4	8	10	13	2	19	8	8	19	43	66	7	13	16
785	**Pears, eating**	N	N	N	N	N	6	10	N	N	N	N	N	N	N	N	N	N	N
786	eating (weighed with skin and core)	N	N	N	N	N	5	7	N	N	N	N	N	N	N	N	N	N	N

Fruit *continued*

Amino acids (mg per 100 g food)

No	Food	Ile	Leu	Lys	Met	Cys	Phe	Tyr	Thr	Trp	Val	Arg	His	Ala	Asp	Glu	Gly	Pro	Ser
787	**Pears, cooking**																		
788	stewed without sugar	N	N	N	N	N	6	10	N	N	N	N	N	N	N	N	N	N	N
789	stewed with sugar	N	N	N	N	N	5	7	N	N	N	N	N	N	N	N	N	N	N
790	canned	N	N	N	N	N	5	7	N	N	N	N	N	N	N	N	N	N	N
791	**Pineapple** fresh	N	N	11	2	N	13	13	N	6	N	N	N	N	N	N	N	N	N
792	canned	N	N	6	1	N	6	6	N	3	N	N	N	N	N	N	N	N	N
809	**Raisins** dried	9	22	24	36	17	22	19	29	5	29	78	39	44	130	220	32	36	51
817	**Strawberries** raw	14	32	25	1	5	18	21	19	7	18	27	12	32	140	92	25	20	24
818	canned	10	22	18	1	4	13	15	13	5	13	19	8	22	98	64	18	14	17
819	**Sultanas** dried	14	36	39	59	28	36	31	48	8	48	130	64	73	210	360	53	59	84
820	**Tangerines** raw	25	24	46	13	11	32	18	13	6	34	56	13	55	120	110	90	49	25
821	raw (weighed with peel and pips)	18	17	33	9	8	23	13	9	4	24	40	9	39	88	76	64	35	18

Nuts

No	Food	Ile	Leu	Lys	Met	Cys	Phe	Tyr	Thr	Trp	Val	Arg	His	Ala	Asp	Glu	Gly	Pro	Ser
822	**Almonds**	720	1280	460	260	290	980	590	490	160	1050	2000	460	790	1930	4480	1080	980	720
823	(weighed with shells)	270	470	170	97	110	360	220	180	61	390	740	170	290	710	1660	400	360	270
824	**Barcelona nuts**	740	800	370	120	140	470	470	370	190	800	1880	250	N	910	2640	1220	720	1240
825	(weighed with shells)	460	500	230	77	90	290	290	230	120	500	1170	150	N	560	1640	760	450	770
826	**Brazil nuts**	400	950	380	800	290	530	380	350	160	600	1830	310	490	1020	2560	620	660	600
827	(weighed with shells)	180	430	170	360	130	240	170	160	69	270	820	140	220	460	1150	280	300	270
830	**Cob** or **hazel nuts**	520	560	260	86	100	330	330	260	130	560	1310	170	N	630	1840	850	500	860
831	(weighed with shells)	190	200	94	31	36	120	120	94	47	200	470	62	N	230	670	310	180	310
832	**Coconut** fresh	150	260	130	67	61	170	100	130	43	210	500	79	170	340	710	170	140	180
834	desiccated	250	440	230	120	110	290	180	220	74	360	860	140	290	580	1230	290	240	320
835	**Peanuts** fresh	950	1800	990	320	360	1400	1080	720	320	1170	3150	680	1080	3200	5130	1580	1220	1350
836	(weighed with shells)	650	1240	680	220	250	960	740	500	220	810	2170	470	740	2200	3530	1090	840	930
837	roasted and salted	950	1800	990	320	360	1400	1080	720	320	1170	3150	680	1080	3200	5130	1580	1220	1350
838	**Peanut butter** smooth	960	1750	880	330	330	1290	880	670	380	1170	3130	630	1170	3170	5170	1500	1210	1500
839	**Walnuts**	500	900	240	180	220	540	420	380	120	600	1580	260	N	N	N	N	N	N
840	(weighed with shells)	320	580	150	120	140	350	270	240	77	380	1010	170	N	N	N	N	N	N

Sugars, preserves, confectionery and beverages

Amino acids (mg per 100 g food)

No	Food	Ile	Leu	Lys	Met	Cys	Phe	Tyr	Thr	Trp	Val	Arg	His	Ala	Asp	Glu	Gly	Pro	Ser
852	**Lemon curd** home made	190	230	210	110	58	170	130	170	58	250	200	80	180	360	400	100	130	260
853	**Marmalade**	2	2	3	1	1	2	1	1	0	2	4	1	4	9	8	6	4	2
854	**Marzipan** almond paste	360	630	230	130	150	490	290	240	81	520	990	230	390	960	2220	540	490	360
857	**Chocolate** milk	540	920	650	220	110	550	270	410	160	590	370	300	380	740	1880	240	890	590
858	plain	180	300	200	90	90	260	98	200	68	270	300	90	220	470	870	200	260	250
868	**Cocoa powder**	670	1070	700	300	370	780	520	700	300	1040	1260	300	810	1780	3030	780	1040	1040
869	**Coffee and chicory essence**	36	83	7	30	10	53	33	26	26	56	0	23	59	96	300	76	56	23
871	**Coffee** infusion, 5 minutes	4	10	1	4	1	6	4	3	3	7	0	3	7	12	36	9	7	3
872	instant	360	820	65	290	98	520	330	260	260	550	0	230	590	950	2970	750	550	230
873	**Drinking chocolate**	190	300	200	83	100	220	150	200	83	290	350	83	230	500	850	220	290	290

Soft drinks and alcoholic beverages

Amino acids (mg per 100 g food)

No	Food	Ile	Leu	Lys	Met	Cys	Phe	Tyr	Thr	Trp	Val	Arg	His	Ala	Asp	Glu	Gly	Pro	Ser
879	**Grapefruit juice** canned, unsweetened	9	9	17	5	4	12	7	5	2	12	20	5	20	44	38	32	18	9
880	sweetened	14	14	26	7	6	18	10	7	3	19	32	7	31	70	61	51	28	14
885	**Orange juice** canned, unsweetened	13	12	23	6	6	16	9	6	3	17	28	6	27	62	53	45	25	13
886	sweetened	20	19	36	10	9	25	14	10	4	26	44	10	43	97	84	70	39	20
887	**Pineapple juice** canned	N	N	7	1	N	8	8	N	4	N	N	N	N	N	N	N	N	N
890	**Tomato juice** canned	14	20	22	5	5	13	10	17	6	16	16	11	18	86	N	13	12	19
	Beers																		
891	**Brown ale** bottled	4	7	6	2	6	6	6	7	8	7	8	5	10	14	42	11	36	8
892	**Canned** bitter	4	7	6	2	6	6	6	7	8	7	8	5	10	14	42	11	36	8
893	**Draught** bitter	4	7	6	2	6	6	6	7	8	7	8	5	10	14	42	11	36	8
894	mild	3	5	4	2	4	4	5	5	6	5	6	4	8	11	32	8	27	6
895	**Keg** bitter	4	7	6	2	6	6	6	7	8	7	8	5	10	14	42	11	36	8
896	**Lager** bottled	3	5	7	2	4	4	5	5	12	5	5	4	8	11	36	9	26	7
897	**Pale ale** bottled	5	9	7	3	7	7	8	9	10	9	10	6	13	18	53	14	45	11
898	**Stout** bottled	5	9	7	3	7	7	8	9	10	9	10	6	13	18	53	14	45	11
899	**Stout** extra	5	9	7	3	7	7	8	9	10	9	10	6	13	18	53	14	45	11
900	**Strong ale**	10	20	15	7	15	15	18	19	21	20	21	13	28	39	120	30	98	23
	Liqueurs																		
916	**Advocaat**	260	390	290	150	83	240	190	240	83	350	290	110	260	500	560	140	180	370

Sauces and pickles, soups and miscellaneous

Amino acids (mg per 100 g food)

No	Food	Ile	Leu	Lys	Met	Cys	Phe	Tyr	Thr	Trp	Val	Arg	His	Ala	Asp	Glu	Gly	Pro	Ser
	Sauces and pickles																		
920	**Bread sauce**	220	400	260	110	57	230	170	180	58	280	170	120	160	310	1160	110	460	250
922	**Cheese sauce**	450	820	630	230	89	440	360	390	120	580	330	240	310	670	1950	190	790	480
923	**Chutney** apple	26	47	44	6	10	19	11	28	7	30	20	14	34	160	84	29	24	32
924	tomato	22	31	32	7	7	20	14	25	9	23	23	16	27	130	N	20	18	29
926	**Mayonnaise**	100	150	110	58	32	93	73	93	32	140	110	44	99	190	220	55	70	140
927	**Onion sauce**	140	260	200	73	34	150	122	130	40	190	130	79	99	210	700	65	270	160
931	**Tomato ketchup**	41	58	61	14	14	37	27	48	17	44	44	31	51	250	N	37	34	54
932	**Tomato purée**	120	170	180	39	39	110	78	140	49	130	130	87	150	700	N	110	97	160
933	**Tomato sauce**	66	110	86	32	27	68	47	55	17	72	78	41	72	110	350	66	120	71
934	**White sauce** savoury	450	820	630	230	90	440	360	390	20	590	330	240	310	670	1970	190	800	490
935	sweet	360	650	360	170	140	390	260	290	97	440	290	190	260	480	2190	210	860	440
	Soup																		
943	**Lentil**	200	350	300	51	49	230	150	180	46	230	330	120	190	470	840	170	250	240
	Miscellaneous																		
956	**Baking powder**	220	400	110	91	150	270	150	160	64	250	200	120	170	250	1880	180	720	320
957	**Bovril**	1000	1810	2060	500	130	1190	690	1380	190	1560	2190	880	3000	2750	4690	4440	3310	1500
959	**Gelatin**	1370	2740	3800	760	0	1980	300	1820	0	2130	7450	610	9270	5620	9580	2950	3070	3500
961	**Marmite**	1920	2380	2850	530	400	1590	730	2050	530	2450	1060	930	2710	3840	5160	2050	1990	2050
968	**Yeast** bakers, compressed	630	910	1030	220	120	550	470	610	140	810	650	360	810	1250	1350	590	530	690
969	dried	1960	2840	3220	700	380	1710	1450	1900	440	2530	2020	1140	2530	3920	4230	1830	1640	2150

The tables
continued

Section 3A
Fatty acid composition
g fatty acids per 100g food

Common names of the most frequently occurring fatty acids

Carbon:	Double bonds	Common name
Saturated		
C4:0		Butyric
C6:0		Caproic
C8:0		Caprylic
C10:0		Capric
C12:0		Lauric
C14:0		Myristic
C16:0		Palmitic
C18:0		Stearic
C20:0		Arachidic
C22:0		Behenic
C24:0		Lignoceric
Mono-unsaturated		
C16:1		Palmitoleic
C18:1		Oleic
C20:1		Eicosenoic
C22:1		Erucic
Polyunsaturated		
C18:2		Linoleic
C18:3		Linolenic
C20:4		Arachidonic

( ) **Estimated value**
N **No information available**
Tr **Trace**

Cereals and cereal products

Fatty acids (g per 100g food)

No	Food	Saturated														
		4:0	6:0	8:0	10:0	12:0	14:0	15:0	16:0	17:0	18:0	20:0	22:0	Total
	Grains, flours and starches													
2	**Barley** pearl, raw	0	0	0	0	0	Tr	0	0.29	0	Tr	0	0	0.29
3	boiled	0	0	0	0	0	Tr	0	0.10	0	Tr	0	0	0.10
4	**Bemax**	0	0	0	0	Tr	Tr	0	1.04	0	0.06	0.05	0	1.15
5	**Bran** wheat	0	0	0	0	0	0	0	0.84	0	0.05	0.04	0	0.93
6	**Cornflour**	0	0	0	0	0	Tr	0	0.09	0	0.02	Tr	0	0.11
7	**Custard powder**	0	0	0	0	0	Tr	0	0.09	0	0.02	Tr	0	0.11
9	**Flour,** wholemeal (100%)	0	0	0	0	0	0	0	0.26	0	0.01	0.01	0	0.28
10	brown (85%)	0	0	0	0	0	0	0	0.26	0	0.01	0.01	0	0.28
11	white (72%) breadmaking	0	0	0	0	0	0	0	0.16	0	Tr	Tr	0	0.16
12	household plain	0	0	0	0	0	0	0	0.16	0	Tr	Tr	0	0.16
13	self-raising	0	0	0	0	0	0	0	0.16	0	Tr	Tr	0	0.16
14	patent (40%)	0	0	0	0	0	0	0	0.17	0	Tr	Tr	0	0.17
15	**Macaroni,** raw	0	0	0	0	0	0	0	0.26	0	0.01	0.01	0	0.28
16	boiled	0	0	0	0	0	0	0	0.08	0	Tr	Tr	0	0.08
17	**Oatmeal** raw	0	0	0	0	0	0	0	1.39	0	0.09	0.04	0	1.52
18	**Porridge**	0	0	0	0	0	0	0	0.14	0	Tr	Tr	0	0.14

Cereals and cereal products *continued*

No	Food	Mono-unsaturated								Polyunsaturated							
		14:1	15:1	16:1	17:1	18:1	20:1	22:1	Total	18:2	18:3	20:4	20:5	22:6	20:1–20:5	22:5 & 22:6	Total
	Grains, flours and starches																
2	**Barley** pearl, raw	0	0	Tr	0	0.14	0	0	0.14	0.70	0.07	0	0	0	0	0	0.77
3	boiled	0	0	Tr	0	0.05	0	0	0.05	0.25	0.03	0	0	0	0	0	0.28
4	**Bemax**	0	0	0.03	0	0.87	0.02	0	0.92	3.37	0.23	0.01	0	0	N	0	3.61
5	**Bran** wheat	0	0	0.02	0	0.69	0.02	0	0.73	2.68	0.18	Tr	0	0	Tr	0	2.86
6	**Cornflour**	0	0	Tr	0	0.20	Tr	Tr	0.20	0.33	0.01	0	0	0	0	0	0.34
7	**Custard powder**	0	0	Tr	0	0.20	Tr	Tr	0.20	0.33	0.01	0	0	0	0	0	0.34
9	**Flour,** wholemeal (100%)	0	0	Tr	0	0.21	Tr	0	0.21	0.83	0.06	Tr	0	0	Tr	0	0.89
10	brown (85%)	0	0	Tr	0	0.21	Tr	0	0.21	0.83	0.06	Tr	0	0	Tr	0	0.89
11	white (72%) breadmaking	0	0	Tr	0	0.13	Tr	0	0.13	0.50	0.03	Tr	0	0	Tr	0	0.53
12	household plain	0	0	Tr	0	0.13	Tr	0	0.13	0.50	0.03	Tr	0	0	Tr	0	0.53
13	self-raising	0	0	Tr	0	0.13	Tr	0	0.13	0.50	0.03	Tr	0	0	Tr	0	0.53
14	patent (40%)	0	0	Tr	0	0.14	Tr	0	0.14	0.54	0.04	Tr	0	0	Tr	0	0.58
15	**Macaroni,** raw	0	0	Tr	0	0.21	Tr	0	0.21	0.83	0.06	Tr	0	0	Tr	0	0.89
16	boiled	0	0	Tr	0	0.06	Tr	0	0.06	0.25	0.02	Tr	0	0	Tr	0	0.27
17	**Oatmeal** raw	0	0	0.02	0	3.14	0	0	3.16	3.33	0.18	0	0	0	0	0	3.51
18	**Porridge**	0	0	Tr	0	0.32	0	0	0.32	0.34	0.02	0	0	0	0	0	0.36

Cereals *continued*

Fatty acids (g per 100g food)

No	Food	Saturated												Total
		4:0	6:0	8:0	10:0	12:0	14:0	15:0	16:0	17:0	18:0	20:0	22:0	
	Grains, flours and starches													
	contd													
19	**Rice** polished, raw	0	0	0	0	0	Tr	0	0.20	0	0.02	Tr	0	0.22
20	boiled	0	0	0	0	0	Tr	0	0.06	0	Tr	Tr	0	0.06
21	**Rye** flour (100%)	0	0	0	0	0	0	0	0.27	0	Tr	0	0	0.27
23	**Semolina** raw	0	0	0	0	0	0	0	0.24	0	0.01	0.01	0	0.26
24	**Soya** flour, full fat	0	0	0	0	0.02	0.04	0	2.25	0	0.90	0.07	0.02	3.30
25	low fat	0	0	0	0	Tr	0.01	0	0.69	0	0.28	0.02	Tr	1.00
26	**Spaghetti** raw	0	0	0	0	0	0	0	0.13	0	Tr	Tr	0	0.13
27	boiled	0	0	0	0	0	0	0	0.04	0	Tr	Tr	0	0.04
	Bread and rolls													
30	**Bread** wholemeal	0	0	0	0	0	0.04	0	0.41	0	0.09	0	0	0.54
31	brown	0	0	0	0	0	0.03	0	0.34	0	0.07	0	0	0.44
32	Hovis	0	0	0	0	0	0.03	0	0.34	0	0.07	0	0	0.44
33	white	0	0	0	0	Tr	0.02	0	0.31	0	0.07	0	0	0.40

Cereals continued

No	Food	Mono-unsaturated								Polyunsaturated							
		14:1	15:1	16:1	17:1	18:1	20:1	22:1	Total	18:2	18:3	20:4	20:5	22:6	20:1 – 20:5	22:5 & 22:6	Total
	Grains, flours and starches *contd*																
19	**Rice** polished, raw	0	0	Tr	0	0.25	0	0	0.25	0.35	Tr	0	0	0	0	0	0.35
20	boiled	0	0	Tr	0	0.08	0	0	0.08	0.11	Tr	0	0	0	0	0	0.11
21	**Rye** flour (100%)	0	0	Tr	0	0.20	0.01	0	0.21	0.82	0.13	0	0	0	0	0	0.95
23	**Semolina** raw	0	0	Tr	0	0.19	Tr	0	0.19	0.75	0.05	Tr	0	0	Tr	0	0.80
24	**Soya** flour, full fat	0	0	0.04	0	5.62	0.04	0	5.70	1.68	1.66	0	0	0	0	0	13.34
25	low fat	0	0	0.01	0	1.72	0.01	0	1.74	3.58	0.51	0	0	0	0	0	4.09
26	**Spaghetti**, raw	0	0	Tr	0	0.11	Tr	0	0.11	0.42	0.03	Tr	0	0	Tr	0	0.45
27	boiled	0	0	Tr	0	0.03	Tr	0	0.03	0.12	Tr	Tr	0	0	Tr	0	0.12
	Bread and rolls																
30	**Bread**, wholemeal	0	0	0.04	0	0.37	0	0	0.41	1.08	0.08	0	0	0	0	0	1.16
31	brown	0	0	0.03	0	0.30	0	0	0.33	0.88	0.06	0	0	0	0	0	0.94
32	Hovis	0	0	0.03	0	0.30	0	0	0.33	0.88	0.06	0	0	0	0	0	0.94
33	white	0	0	0.01	0	0.24	0	0	0.25	0.62	0.04	0	0	0	0	0	0.66

Cereals continued

Fatty acids (g per 100g food)

No	Food	Saturated												Total
		4:0	6:0	8:0	10:0	12:0	14:0	15:0	16:0	17:0	18:0	20:0	22:0	
	Bread contd													
35	white, toasted	0	0	0	0	Tr	0.02	0	0.31	0	0.07	0	0	0.40
36	dried crumbs	0	0	0	0	0.01	0.02	0	0.35	0	0.08	0	0	0.46
37	currant	0	0	0	0	0.02	0.04	0	0.63	0	0.14	0	0	0.83
39	soda	0.05	0.03	0.02	0.04	0.05	0.16	0.02	0.47	0.01	0.16	Tr	0	1.01
40	**Rolls** brown, crusty	0	0	0	0	0	0.04	0	0.49	0	0.11	0	0	0.64
41	soft	0	0	0	0	0	0.09	0	0.98	0	0.22	0	0	1.29
42	white, crusty	0	0	0	0	0.02	0.04	0	0.59	0	0.13	0	0	0.78
43	soft	0	0	0	0	0.04	0.09	0	1.34	0	0.29	0	0	1.76
44	starch reduced	0	0	0	0	0	0	0	0.54	0	0.03	0.02	0	0.59
46	**Chapatis** made without fat	0	0	0	0	0	0	0	0.13	0	Tr	Tr	0	0.13
	Breakfast cereals													
47	**All-bran**	0	0	0	0	0	0	0	0.87	0	0.05	0.04	0	0.96
48	**Cornflakes**	0	0	0	0	0	Tr	0	0.21	0	0.04	Tr	0	0.25
50	**Muesli**	0	0	0	0	0	0	0	1.20	0	0.08	0.04	0	1.32
51	**Puffed Wheat**	0	0	0	0	0	0	0	0.17	0	Tr	Tr	0	0.17
52	**Ready Brek**	0	0	0	0	0	0	0	1.39	0	0.09	0.04	0	1.52
53	**Rice Krispies**	0	0	0	0	0	0.02	0	0.41	0	0.04	Tr	0	0.47

Cereals *continued*

No	Food	Mono-unsaturated								Polyunsaturated							
		14:1	15:1	16:1	17:1	18:1	20:1	22:1	Total	18:2	18:3	20:4	20:5	22:6	20:1–20:5	22:5 & 22:6	Total
	Bread *contd*																
35	white toasted	0	0	0.01	0	0.24	0	0	0.25	0.62	0.04	0	0	0	0	0	0.66
36	dried crumbs	0	0	0.02	0	0.27	0	0	0.29	0.69	0.05	0	0	0	0	0	0.74
37	currant	0	0	0.03	0	0.48	0	0	0.51	1.23	0.09	0	0	0	0	0	1.32
39	soda	0.02	Tr	0.04	0.02	0.48	Tr	0	0.56	0.36	0.04	Tr	0	0	Tr	0	0.40
40	**Rolls** brown, crusty	0	0	0.05	0	0.43	0	0	0.43	1.29	0.09	0	0	0	0	0	1.38
41	soft	0	0	0.10	0	0.87	0	0	0.97	2.57	0.18	0	0	0	0	0	2.75
42	white, crusty	0	0	0.03	0	0.45	0	0	0.43	1.16	0.08	0	0	0	0	0	1.24
43	soft	0	0	0.06	0	1.03	0	0	1.09	2.65	0.19	0	0	0	0	0	2.84
44	starch reduced	0	0	0.01	0	0.44	0.01	0	0.46	1.70	0.12	Tr	0	0	Tr	0	1.82
46	**Chapatis** made without fat	0	0	Tr	0	0.11	Tr	0	0.11	0.42	0.03	Tr	0	0	Tr	0	0.45
	Breakfast cereals																
47	**All-bran**	0	0	0.02	0	0.72	0.02	0	0.76	2.78	0.19	Tr	0	0	Tr	0	2.97
48	**Cornflakes**	0	0	Tr	0	0.46	Tr	Tr	0.46	0.76	0.02	0	0	0	0	0	0.78
50	**Muesli**	0	0	0.01	0	2.71	0	0	2.72	2.87	0.16	0	0	0	0	0	3.03
51	**Puffed Wheat**	0	0	Tr	0	0.14	Tr	0	0.14	0.54	0.04	Tr	0	0	Tr	0	0.58
52	**Ready Brek**	0	0	0.02	0	3.14	0	0	3.16	3.33	0.18	0	0	0	0	0	3.51
53	**Rice Krispies**	0	0	Tr	0	0.50	0	0	0.50	0.70	0.02	0	0	0	0	0	0.72

Cereals *continued*

Fatty acids (g per 100g food)

No	Food	Saturated												Total
		4:0	6:0	8:0	10:0	12:0	14:0	15:0	16:0	17:0	18:0	20:0	22:0	
	Breakfast cereals *contd*													
54	**Shredded Wheat**	0	0	0	0	0	0	0	0.39	0	0.02	0.02	0	0.43
56	**Sugar Puffs**	0	0	0	0	0	0	0	0.10	0	Tr	Tr	0	0.10
57	**Weetabix**	0	0	0	0	0	0	0	0.45	0	0.02	0.02	0	0.49
	Biscuits													
58	**Chocolate** full coated[a]	0	0	0	0.26	2.81	1.34	0	6.74	0	5.27	0.13	0	16.55
60	**Crispbread** rye	0	0	0	0	Tr	Tr	0	0.28	0	0.01	0	0	0.29
61	wheat, starch reduced[a]	0	0	0	0	0.04	0.06	0	2.34	0	0.24	0.01	0	2.69
63	**Digestive** chocolate[a]	0	0	0	0	0.14	0.50	0	7.12	0	4.05	0.21	0	12.02
64	**Ginger nuts**[a]	0	0	0	0	0.16	0.40	0	5.17	0	1.33	0.09	0	7.15
65	**Home made**	0	0	0	0	0.06	1.11	0	4.16	0.19	1.60	0.39	0.38	7.89
66	**Matzo**	0	0	0	0	0.01	Tr	0	0.28	0	Tr	0	0	0.29
67	**Oatcakes**[a]	0	0	0	0	0.05	0.33	0	2.68	0	0.75	0.10	0	3.91
68	**Sandwich**[a]	0	0	0.34	0.37	3.44	1.45	0	6.62	0	2.09	0.10	0	14.41
69	**Semi-sweet**[a]	0	0	0	0	0.35	0.49	0	5.60	0	1.39	0.09	0	7.92
70	**Short-sweet**[a]	0	0	0	0	0.67	0.84	0	8.11	0	1.82	0.20	0	11.64
71	**Shortbread**	0.77	0.48	0.29	0.67	0.84	2.68	0.26	6.31	0.24	2.68	Tr	0	15.22
72	**Wafers** filled[a]	0	0	0.97	0.80	8.15	2.98	0	4.09	0	1.45	0	0	18.44

[a] The composition may vary according to type of fat used in the manufacture of these foods

Cereals *continued*

Fatty acids (g per 100g food)

No	Food	Mono-unsaturated								Polyunsaturated							
		14:1	15:1	16:1	17:1	18:1	20:1	22:1	Total	18:2	18:3	20:4	20:5	22:6	20:1 – 20:5	22:5 & 22:6	Total
	Breakfast cereals *contd*																
54	**Shredded Wheat**	0	0	0.01	0	0.32	Tr	0	0.33	1.25	0.09	Tr	0	0	Tr	0	1.34
56	**Sugar Puffs**	0	0	Tr	0	0.09	Tr	0	0.09	0.33	0.02	Tr	0	0	Tr	0	0.35
57	**Weetabix**	0	0	0.01	0	0.36	Tr	0	0.37	1.41	0.10	Tr	0	0	Tr	0	1.51
	Biscuits																
58	**Chocolate** full coated[a]	0	0	0.18	0	7.71	0.08	0	7.97	1.08	0.05	0	0	0	0	0	1.13
60	**Crispbread** rye	0	0	Tr	0	0.22	0.02	0	0.24	0.85	0.11	0	0	0	0	0	0.96
61	wheat, starch reduced[a]	0	0	0.02	0	1.98	0.04	0	2.04	2.36	0.12	0	0	0	0	0	2.48
63	**Digestive** chocolate[a]	0	0	0.23	0	8.06	0.37	0.23	8.89	1.51	0.05	0	0	0	0	0	1.56
64	**Ginger nuts**[a]	0	0	0.23	0	5.29	0.14	0.12	5.78	1.31	0.07	0	0	0	0	0	1.38
65	**Home made**	0	0	1.16	0	4.69	1.63	1.68	9.16	1.26	0.06	0.28	1.11	0.01	N	0.76	3.48
66	**Matzo**	0	0	Tr	0	0.14	0.01	0	0.15	0.86	0.05	0	0	0	0	0	0.91
67	**Oatcakes**[a]	0	0	0.24	0	6.62	0.73	0.54	8.13	4.73	0.42	0	0	0	0	0	5.15
68	**Sandwich**[a]	0	0	0.17	0	7.63	N	0.12	8.04	1.48	0	N	0	0	0.27	0	1.75
69	**Semi-sweet**[a]	0	0	0.19	0	5.61	N	0.08	5.96	1.48	0	N	0	0	0.22	0	1.70
70	**Short-sweet**[a]	0	0	0.31	0	7.56	N	0	7.98	1.82	0.11	N	0	0	0.49	0	2.42
71	**Shortbread**	0.33	0.17	0.65	0.26	6.72	Tr	0	8.13	0.63	0.38	0	0	0	0	0	1.01
72	**Wafers** filled[a]	0	0	0.09	0	8.10	0	0	8.19	0.88	0	0	0	0	0	0	0.88

[a] The composition may vary according to type of fat used in the manufacture of these foods

Cereals *continued*

Fatty acids (g per 100g food)

No	Food	Saturated												Total
		4:0	6:0	8:0	10:0	12:0	14:0	15:0	16:0	17:0	18:0	20:0	22:0	
	Cakes													
74	**Fancy iced cakes**[a]	0	0	0.35	0.30	3.06	1.33	0	2.56	0	1.68	0	0	9.28
75	**Fruit cake**, rich	0	0	0	0	0.03	0.53	0	2.11	0.09	0.81	0.18	0.18	3.93
76	rich, iced	0	0	0	0	0.02	0.36	0	1.69	0.06	0.62	0.13	0.12	3.00
77	plain[a]	0	0	0	0	0.06	0.64	0	3.75	0	1.23	0.10	0	5.78
78	**Gingerbread**	0.01	Tr	Tr	0.01	0.04	0.62	Tr	2.43	0.10	0.93	0.20	0.20	4.54
79	**Madeira cake**[a]	0	0	0.27	0.26	1.62	1.33	0	3.64	0	1.46	0.11	0.10	8.79
80	**Rock cakes**	Tr	Tr	Tr	Tr	0.05	0.84	Tr	3.10	0.14	1.20	0.28	0.28	5.89
81	**Sponge cake**, with fat	0	0	0	Tr	0.11	1.29	0	5.14	0.22	2.03	0.44	0.44	9.67
82	without fat	0	0	0	0	0	0	0	1.56	0	0.50	Tr	0	2.06
83	jam filled[a]	0	0	0	0	0	0.16	0	1.20	0	0.47	0.04	0	1.87
	Buns and pastries													
86	**Eclairs**	0.41	0.26	0.15	0.36	0.48	1.80	0.14	5.55	0.18	2.88	0.12	0.11	12.44
87	**Jam tarts**	0	0	0	0	0.02	0.48	0	3.32	0.08	1.68	0.13	0.12	5.83
88	**Mince pies**	0	0	0	0	0.02	0.61	0	4.56	0.10	2.17	0.16	0.16	7.78

[a] The composition may vary according to the type of fat used in the manufacture of these foods

Cereals *continued*

No	Food	Mono-unsaturated								Polyunsaturated							
		14:1	15:1	16:1	17:1	18:1	20:1	22:1	Total	18:2	18:3	20:4	20:5	22:6	20:1 – 20:5	22:5 & 22:6	Total
	Cakes																
74	**Fancy Iced cakes**[a]	0	0	0.37	0	2.90	0.23	0.44	3.94	0.72	0.10	0	0	0	0	0	0.82
75	**Fruit cake** rich	0	0	0.57	0	2.44	0.77	0.80	4.58	0.62	0.02	0.13	0.53	0.01	N	0.36	1.67
76	rich, iced	0	0	0.41	0	4.40	0.52	0.54	5.87	1.15	0.03	0.10	0.35	Tr	N	0.24	1.87
77	plain[a]	0	0	0.78	0	3.60	0.49	0.29	5.16	1.04	0.09	0	0	0	0	0	1.13
78	**Gingerbread**	Tr	Tr	0.64	Tr	2.79	0.85	0.87	5.15	0.76	0.04	0.14	0.58	0.01	N	0.40	1.93
79	**Madeira cake**[a]	0	0	0.79	0	3.66	0.45	0.74	5.64	1.46	0	0	0	0	0	0	1.46
80	**Rock cakes**	Tr	Tr	0.85	Tr	3.49	1.19	1.23	6.76	0.90	0.04	0.20	0.81	Tr	N	0.56	2.51
81	**Spongecake** with fat	0	0	1.39	0	5.96	1.87	1.93	11.15	1.31	0.04	0.32	1.28	0.03	N	0.88	3.86
82	without fat	0	0	0.22	0	2.31	0	0	2.53	0.71	Tr	0.04	0	0.06	N	N	0.81
83	jam filled[a]	0	0	0.21	0	1.21	0.15	0.34	1.91	0.65	0.13	0	0	0	0	0	0.78
	Buns and pastries																
86	**Eclairs**	0.18	0.09	0.72	0.14	6.26	0.47	0.49	8.35	0.75	0.21	0.09	0.32	0.02	N	0.22	1.61
87	**Jam tarts**	0	0	0.55	0	4.50	0.59	0.55	6.19	1.12	0.08	0.09	0.36	0	N	0.25	1.90
88	**Mince Pies**	0	0	0.69	0	5.75	0.74	0.69	7.87	2.26	0.28	0.11	0.45	0	N	0.31	3.41

[a]The composition may vary according to the type of fat used in the manufacture of these foods

Cereals *continued*

No	Food	Saturated												Total
		4:0	6:0	8:0	10:0	12:0	14:0	15:0	16:0	17:0	18:0	20:0	22:0	
	Buns and pastries *contd*													
89	**Pastry** choux, raw	0	0	0	0	0.03	0.55	0	2.55	0.10	0.96	0.19	0.19	4.57
90	cooked	0	0	0	0	0.04	0.85	0	3.95	0.15	1.48	0.30	0.29	7.06
91	flaky, raw	0	0	0	0	0.04	1.01	0	6.84	0.16	3.48	0.26	0.26	12.05
92	cooked	0	0	0	0	0.05	1.32	0	8.93	0.21	4.53	0.35	0.34	15.73
93	shortcrust, raw	0	0	0	0	0.03	0.90	0	6.19	0.14	3.14	0.24	0.23	10.87
94	cooked	0	0	0	0	0.04	1.05	0	7.18	0.17	3.64	0.27	0.27	12.62
95	**Scones**	0.05	0.03	0.02	0.04	0.08	0.85	0.02	2.78	0.13	1.09	0.24	0.24	5.57
96	**Scotch pancakes**	0.05	0.03	0.02	0.04	0.08	0.63	0.02	2.29	0.10	0.88	0.16	0.16	4.46
	Puddings													
97	**Apple crumble**	0	0	0	0	0.02	0.37	0	1.28	0.06	0.50	0.13	0.13	2.49
98	**Bread and butter pudding**	0.17	0.11	0.06	0.15	0.19	0.61	0.06	1.89	0.05	0.76	0	0	4.05
99	**Cheesecake**	0.73	0.46	0.27	0.64	0.88	3.00	0.25	8.49	0.29	3.39	0.14	0.12	18.66
100	**Christmas pudding**	0	0	0	0	Tr	0.27	0.04	2.73	0.10	2.30	Tr	0	5.44
101	**Custard,** egg	0.11	0.07	0.04	0.10	0.13	0.40	0.04	1.46	0.04	0.57	0	0	2.96
102	made with powder	0.13	0.08	0.05	0.12	0.15	0.47	0.05	1.08	0.04	0.47	0	0	2.64
103	**Custard tart**	0.06	0.04	0.02	0.05	0.08	0.65	0.02	3.82	0.09	1.84	0.12	0.12	6.91
104	**Dumpling**	0	0	0	0	0	0.36	0.05	3.06	0.13	2.88	Tr	0	6.48

Cereals *continued*

No	Food	Mono-unsaturated								Polyunsaturated					20:1–	22:5 &	
		14:1	15:1	16:1	17:1	18:1	20:1	22:1	Total	18:2	18:3	20:4	20:5	22:6	20:5	22:6	Total
	Buns and pastries *contd*																
89	**Pastry** choux, raw	0	0	0.65	0	3.06	0.81	0.84	5.36	0.81	0.03	0.16	0.55	0.03	N	0.38	1.96
90	cooked	0	0	1.00	0	4.73	1.25	1.30	8.28	1.27	0.04	0.24	0.85	0.04	N	0.59	3.03
91	flaky, raw	0	0	1.15	0	9.28	1.23	1.14	12.80	2.18	0.17	0.19	0.75	0	N	0.52	3.81
92	cooked	0	0	1.51	0	12.10	1.62	1.51	16.74	2.86	0.22	0.24	0.99	0	N	0.68	4.99
93	shortcrust, raw	0	0	1.03	0	8.39	1.11	1.03	11.56	2.07	0.16	0.16	0.68	0	N	0.47	3.54
94	cooked	0	0	1.20	0	9.73	1.28	1.19	13.40	2.39	0.18	0.19	0.78	0	N	0.54	4.08
95	**Scones**	0.02	Tr	0.73	0.02	3.03	1.01	1.04	5.85	0.86	0.06	0.17	0.68	0	N	0.47	2.24
96	**Scotch pancakes**	0.02	0.01	0.54	0.02	2.60	0.68	0.71	4.58	0.70	0.05	0.12	0.47	0.01	N	0.32	1.67
	Puddings																
97	**Apple crumble**	0	0	0.37	0	1.40	0.54	0.56	2.87	0.38	0.02	0.09	0.37	0	N	0.26	1.12
98	**Bread and butter pudding**	0.08	0.04	0.21	0.06	2.20	0	0	2.59	0.32	0.09	0.01	0	0.02	N	N	0.44
99	**Cheesecake**	0.32	0.16	1.04	0.25	9.17	0.53	0.55	12.02	0.99	0.36	0.09	0.35	0.01	0.04	0.24	2.08
100	**Christmas pudding**	0	0.05	0.23	0.13	4.20	0	0	4.61	0.65	0.02	Tr	0	0.01	Tr	N	0.68
101	**Custard,** egg	0.05	0.03	0.17	0.04	1.78	0	0	2.07	0.25	0.05	0.01	0	0.02	N	N	0.33
102	made with powder	0.06	0.03	0.11	0.05	1.16	0	0	1.4	0.06	0.06	0	0	0	0	0	0.12
103	**Custard tart**	0.03	0.01	0.60	0.02	5.07	0.55	0.51	6.79	1.18	0.10	0.09	0.34	0.01	N	0.23	1.95
104	**Dumpling**	0	0.06	0.24	0.17	3.75	Tr	0	4.22	0.31	0.01	0	0	0	0	0	0.32

Fatty acids (g per 100 g food)

No	Food	Saturated												Total
		4:0	6:0	8:0	10:0	12:0	14:0	15:0	16:0	17:0	18:0	20:0	22:0	
	Puddings contd													
106	**Fruit pie** with pastry top	0	0	0	0	Tr	0.24	0	1.69	0.04	0.86	0.06	0.06	2.95
107	**Ice cream**, dairy	0.18	0.12	0.07	0.17	0.23	0.67	0.07	1.98	0.03	0.77	0	0	4.29
108	non-dairy[a]	0	0	0	0	0	0.20	0	3.39	0	0.60	0	0	4.19
111	**Jelly** made with milk	0.05	0.03	0.02	0.04	0.05	0.17	0.02	0.39	0.02	0.17	0.13		0.96
112	**Lemon meringue pie**	0	0	0	0	0.02	0.46	0	3.20	0.08	1.48	0.13	0.13	5.50
114	**Milk pudding**	0.13	0.08	0.05	0.11	0.14	0.44	0.04	1.03	0.04	0.44	0	0	2.50
115	canned, rice	0.13	0.08	0.05	0.11	0.14	0.44	0.04	1.03	0.04	0.44	0	0	2.50
116	**Pancakes**	0.07	0.04	0.02	0.06	0.07	0.42	0.02	4.09	0.04	2.19	Tr	0	7.02
117	**Queen of puddings**	0.17	0.11	0.06	0.15	0.19	0.61	0.06	1.91	0.05	0.77	0	0	4.08
118	**Sponge pudding** steamed	Tr	Tr	Tr	Tr	0.05	0.80	Tr	3.16	0.13	1.21	0.27	0.26	5.88
119	**Suet pudding** steamed	0.03	0.02	0.01	0.03	0.04	0.64	0.09	4.73	0.20	4.30	Tr	0	10.09
120	**Treacle tart**	0	0	0	0	0.02	0.45	0	3.11	0.07	1.56	0.12	0.12	5.45
121	**Trifle**	0.13	0.08	0.05	0.11	0.14	0.44	0.04	1.30	0.04	0.53	Tr	0	2.86
122	**Yorkshire pudding**	0.08	0.05	0.03	0.07	0.09	0.45	0.06	2.50	0.09	1.09	Tr	0	4.51

[a] The composition may vary according to the type of fat used in the manufacture of this food

Fatty acids (g per 100 g food)

No	Food	Mono-unsaturated								Polyunsaturated							
		14:1	15:1	16:1	17:1	18:1	20:1	22:1	Total	18:2	18:3	20:4	20:5	22:6	20:1 – 20:5	22:5 & 22:6	Total
	Puddings contd																
106	**Fruit pie** with pastry top	0	0	0.28	0	2.30	0.30	0.28	3.16	0.57	0.04	0.05	0.18	0	N	0.13	0.97
107	**Ice cream,** dairy	0.05	0	0.11	0.06	1.48	0	0	1.70	0.10	0.06	0	0	0	0	0	0.16
108	non-dairy[a]	0	0	0.06	0	2.74	0.13	0.09	3.02	0.56	0	0	0	0	0	0	0.56
111	**Jelly** made with milk	0.02	0.01	0.04	0.02	0.42	0	0	0.51	0.02	0.02	0	0	0	0	0	0.04
112	**Lemon meringue pie**	0	0	0.58	0	4.29	0.59	0.57	6.03	1.06	0.06	0.10	0.38	0.02	N	0.26	1.88
114	**Milk pudding**	0.06	0.03	0.11	0.04	1.10	0	0	1.34	0.06	0.06	0	0	0	0	0	0.12
115	canned, rice	0.06	0.03	0.11	0.04	1.10	0	0	1.34	0.06	0.06	0	0	0	0	0	0.12
116	**Pancakes**	0.03	0.01	0.40	0.02	5.93	0.09	0	6.48	1.31	0.13	Tr	0	0.01	Tr	N	1.45
117	**Queen of puddings**	0.08	0.04	0.22	0.06	2.24	0	0	2.64	0.33	0.09	0.01	0	0.02	N	N	0.45
118	**Sponge pudding** steamed	Tr	Tr	0.84	Tr	3.65	1.12	1.16	6.77	0.95	0.04	0.19	0.77	0.02	N	0.53	2.50
119	**Suet pudding** steamed	0.01	0.10	0.38	0.26	5.74	0	0	6.49	0.45	0.03	0	0	0	0	0	0.48
120	**Treacle tart**	0	0	0.52	0	4.19	0.55	0.51	5.77	1.09	0.08	0.08	0.34	0	N	0.23	1.82
121	**Trifle**	0.06	0.03	0.14	0.04	2.10	0	0	2.37	0.32	0.06	Tr	0	Tr	Tr	Tr	0.38
122	**Yorkshire pudding**	0.11	0.02	0.46	0.08	3.52	0	0	4.19	0.41	0.11	0.06	0	0.02	N	N	0.60

[a]The composition may vary according to the type of fat used in the manufacture of this food

Milk and milk products

Fatty acids (g per 100 g food)

No	Food	Saturated												Total
		4:0	6:0	8:0	10:0	12:0	14:0	15:0	16:0	17:0	18:0	20:0	22:0	
	Milk, cows'													
124	fresh, whole, summer	0.11	0.07	0.04	0.10	0.13	0.40	0.04	0.93	0.04	0.40	0	0	2.26
125	winter	0.11	0.07	0.04	0.10	0.13	0.40	0.04	0.93	0.04	0.40	0	0	2.26
127	fresh, whole, Channel Isles, summer	0.15	0.09	0.05	0.13	0.16	0.51	0.05	1.18	0.05	0.51	0	0	2.88
128	winter	0.15	0.09	0.05	0.13	0.16	0.51	0.05	1.18	0.05	0.51	0	0	2.88
129	sterilized	0.11	0.07	0.04	0.10	0.13	0.40	0.04	0.93	0.04	0.40	0	0	2.26
130	longlife (UHT treated)	0.11	0.07	0.04	0.10	0.13	0.40	0.04	0.93	0.04	0.40	0	0	2.26
131	fresh, skimmed	Tr	Tr	Tr	Tr	Tr	0.01	Tr	0.02	Tr	0.01	0	0	0.04
132	condensed whole sweetened	0.27	0.17	0.10	0.24	0.30	0.95	0.09	2.21	0.09	0.95	0	0	5.37
133	skimmed, sweetened	Tr	Tr	Tr	Tr	Tr	0.03	Tr	0.07	Tr	0.03	0	0	0.13
134	evaporated, whole, unsweetened	0.27	0.17	0.10	0.24	0.30	0.95	0.09	2.21	0.09	0.95	0	0	5.37
135	dried whole	0.80	0.50	0.30	0.70	0.87	2.78	0.27	6.46	0.25	2.78	0	0	15.71
136	skimmed	0.04	0.02	0.01	0.03	0.04	0.14	0.01	0.32	0.01	0.14	0	0	0.76
137	**Milk goats'**	0.09	0.10	0.14	0.39	0.19	0.48	0	1.15	0	0.41	0	0	2.95
138	**Milk human** mature	0	0	0	0.05	0.21	0.29	0	1.04	0	0.37	0	0	1.96
139	transitional	0	0	0	0.05	0.19	0.26	0	0.94	0	0.34	0	0	1.78
140	**Butter** salted	2.48	1.55	0.93	2.17	2.71	8.68	0.85	20.15	0.77	8.68	0	0	48.97

Milk and milk products *continued*

No	Food	Mono-unsaturated								Polyunsaturated							
		14:1	15:1	16:1	17:1	18:1	20:1	22:1	Total	18:2	18:3	20:4	20:5	22:6	20:1–20:5	22:5 & 22:6	Total
	Milk, cows'																
124	fresh, whole, summer	0.05	0.03	0.10	0.04	1.00	0	0	1.22	0.05	0.05	0	0	0	0	0	0.10
125	winter	0.05	0.03	0.10	0.04	1.00	0	0	1.22	0.05	0.05	0	0	0	0	0	0.10
127	fresh, whole, Channel Isles, summer	0.06	0.03	0.12	0.05	1.26	0	0	1.52	0.06	0.07	0	0	0	0	0	0.13
128	winter	0.06	0.03	0.12	0.05	1.26	0	0	1.52	0.06	0.07	0	0	0	0	0	0.13
129	sterilized	0.05	0.03	0.10	0.04	1.00	0	0	1.22	0.05	0.05	0	0	0	0	0	0.10
130	longlife (UHT treated)	0.05	0.03	0.10	0.04	1.00	0	0	1.22	0.05	0.05	0	0	0	0	0	0.10
131	fresh, skimmed	Tr	Tr	Tr	Tr	0.03	0	0	0.03	Tr	Tr	0	0	0	0	0	0.00
132	condensed, whole, sweetened	0.12	0.06	0.23	0.09	2.36	0	0	2.86	0.12	0.13	0	0	0	0	0	0.25
133	skimmed, sweetened	Tr	Tr	Tr	Tr	0.08	0	0	0.08	Tr	Tr	0	0	0	0	0	0.00
134	evaporated, whole, unsweetened	0.12	0.06	0.23	0.09	2.36	0	0	2.86	0.12	0.13	0	0	0	0	0	0.25
135	dried, whole	0.35	0.17	0.67	0.27	6.91	0	0	8.37	0.35	0.37	0	0	0	0	0	0.72
136	skimmed	0.02	Tr	0.03	0.01	0.34	0	0	0.40	0.02	0.02	0	0	0	0	0	0.04
137	**Milk goats'**	0	0	0.10	0	1.11	0	0	1.21	0.10	(0.04)	0	0	0	0	0	0.14
138	**Milk human** mature	0	0	0.16	0.02	1.39	0.02	0	1.59	0.28	0.03	0	0	0	0	0	0.31
139	transitional	0	0	0.14	0.02	1.25	0.02	0	1.43	0.25	0.03	0	0	0	0	0	0.28
140	**Butter** salted	1.08	0.54	2.09	0.85	21.54	0	0	26.10	1.08	1.16	0	0	0	0	0	2.24

Milk and milk products *continued*

Fatty acids (g per 100 g food)

No	Food	Saturated												Total
		4:0	6:0	8:0	10:0	12:0	14:0	15:0	16:0	17:0	18:0	20:0	22:0	
	Cream													
142	single, summer	0.64	0.40	0.24	0.56	0.70	2.24	0.22	5.21	0.20	2.24	0	0	12.65
143	winter	0.64	0.40	0.24	0.56	0.70	2.24	0.22	5.21	0.20	2.24	0	0	12.65
145	double, summer	1.46	0.91	0.55	1.28	1.59	5.10	0.50	11.84	0.46	5.10	0	0	28.79
146	winter	1.46	0.91	0.55	1.28	1.59	5.10	0.50	11.84	0.46	5.10	0	0	28.79
148	whipping, summer	1.06	0.66	0.40	0.93	1.16	3.70	0.36	8.60	0.33	3.70	0	0	20.90
149	winter	1.06	0.66	0.40	0.93	1.16	3.70	0.36	8.60	0.33	3.70	0	0	20.90
150	sterilized, canned	0.70	0.44	0.26	0.62	0.77	2.47	0.24	5.72	0.22	2.47	0	0	13.91
	Cheese													
151	Camembert type	0.70	0.44	0.26	0.61	0.77	2.46	0.24	5.70	0.22	2.46	0	0	13.86
152	Cheddar type	1.01	0.63	0.38	0.89	1.11	3.55	0.35	8.23	0.32	3.55	0	0	20.02
153	Danish Blue type	0.88	0.55	0.33	0.77	0.97	3.09	0.30	7.17	0.28	3.09	0	0	17.43
154	Edam type	0.69	0.43	0.26	0.61	0.76	2.42	0.24	5.63	0.22	2.42	0	0	13.68
155	Parmesan	0.90	0.56	0.34	0.79	0.98	3.14	0.31	7.30	0.28	3.14	0	0	17.74
156	Stilton	1.21	0.76	0.45	1.06	1.32	4.23	0.42	9.83	0.38	4.23	0	0	23.89
157	cottage cheese†	0.12	0.08	0.05	0.11	0.13	0.42	0.04	0.98	0.04	0.42	0	0	2.39
158	cream cheese	1.43	0.90	0.54	1.25	1.57	5.02	0.49	11.65	0.45	5.02	0	0	28.32
159	processed cheese	0.76	0.47	0.28	0.66	0.83	2.65	0.26	6.14	0.24	2.65	0	0	14.94
160	cheese spread	0.69	0.43	0.26	0.61	0.76	2.42	0.24	5.63	0.22	2.42	0	0	13.68
	Yogurt low fat													
161	natural	0.03	0.02	0.01	0.03	0.03	0.11	0.01	0.25	Tr	0.11	0	0	0.60
162	flavoured	0.03	0.02	0.01	0.02	0.03	0.10	Tr	0.22	Tr	0.10	0	0	0.53
163	fruit	0.03	0.02	0.01	0.03	0.03	0.11	0.01	0.25	Tr	0.11	0	0	0.60
164	hazelnut	0.08	0.05	0.03	0.07	0.09	0.28	0.03	0.64	0.02	0.28	0	0	1.57

†see footnote on p 75 of 'The Composition of Foods'

Milk and milk products _continued_

Fatty acids (g per 100 g food)

No	Food	Mono-unsaturated								Polyunsaturated							
		14:1	15:1	16:1	17:1	18:1	20:1	22:1	Total	18:2	18:3	20:4	20:5	22:6	20:1 – 20:5	22:5 & 22:6	Total
	Cream																
142	single, summer	0.28	0.14	0.54	0.22	5.57	0	0	6.75	0.28	0.30	0	0	0	0	0	0.58
143	winter	0.28	0.14	0.54	0.22	5.57	0	0	6.75	0.28	0.30	0	0	0	0	0	0.58
145	double, summer	0.64	0.32	1.23	0.50	12.66	0	0	15.35	0.64	0.68	0	0	0	0	0	1.32
146	winter	0.64	0.32	1.23	0.50	12.66	0	0	15.35	0.64	0.68	0	0	0	0	0	1.32
148	whipping, summer	0.46	0.23	0.89	0.36	9.19	0	0	11.13	0.46	0.50	0	0	0	0	0	0.96
149	winter	0.46	0.23	0.89	0.36	9.19	0	0	11.13	0.46	0.50	0	0	0	0	0	0.96
150	sterilized, canned	0.31	0.15	0.59	0.24	6.12	0	0	7.41	0.31	0.33	0	0	0	0	0	0.64
	Cheese																
151	Camembert type	0.31	0.15	0.59	0.24	6.09	0	0	7.38	0.31	0.33	0	0	0	0	0	0.64
152	Cheddar type	0.44	0.22	0.85	0.35	8.80	0	0	10.66	0.44	0.47	0	0	0	0	0	0.91
153	Danish Blue type	0.39	0.19	0.75	0.30	7.67	0	0	9.30	0.39	0.41	0	0	0	0	0	0.80
154	Edam type	0.30	0.15	0.58	0.24	6.02	0	0	7.29	0.30	0.32	0	0	0	0	0	0.62
155	Parmesan	0.39	0.20	0.76	0.31	7.80	0	0	9.46	0.39	0.42	0	0	0	0	0	0.81
156	Stilton	0.53	0.26	1.02	0.42	10.51	0	0	12.74	0.53	0.57	0	0	0	0	0	1.10
157	cottage cheese†	0.05	0.03	0.10	0.04	1.05	0	0	1.27	0.05	0.06	0	0	0	0	0	0.11
158	cream cheese	0.63	0.31	1.21	0.49	12.45	0	0	15.09	0.63	0.67	0	0	0	0	0	1.30
159	processed cheese	0.33	0.17	0.64	0.26	6.57	0	0	7.97	0.33	0.35	0	0	0	0	0	0.68
160	cheese spread	0.30	0.15	0.58	0.24	6.02	0	0	7.29	0.30	0.32	0	0	0	0	0	0.62
	Yogurt low fat																
161	natural	0.01	Tr	0.03	0.01	0.26	0	0	0.31	0.01	0.01	0	0	0	0	0	0.02
162	flavoured	0.01	Tr	0.02	Tr	0.24	0	0	0.27	0.01	0.01	0	0	0	0	0	0.02
163	fruit	0.01	Tr	0.03	0.01	0.26	0	0	0.31	0.01	0.01	0	0	0	0	0	0.02
164	hazelnut	0.03	0.02	0.07	0.03	0.68	0	0	0.83	0.03	0.04	0	0	0	0	0	0.07

†see footnote on p 75 of 'The Composition of Foods'

No	Food	Saturated												Total
		4:0	6:0	8:0	10:0	12:0	14:0	15:0	16:0	17:0	18:0	20:0	22:0	
	Eggs													
165	Whole raw	0	0	0	0	0	0	0	2.59	0	0.84	0	0	3.43
167	Yolk raw	0	0	0	0	0	0	0	7.24	0	2.35	0	0	9.59
168	Dried	0	0	0	0	0	0	0	10.28	0	3.34	0	0	13.62
169	Boiled	0	0	0	0	0	0	0	2.59	0	0.84	0	0	3.43
171	Poached	0	0	0	0	0	0	0	2.78	0	0.90	0	0	3.68
172	Omelette	0.11	0.07	0.04	0.09	0.12	0.37	0.04	3.16	0.03	1.12	0	0	5.15
173	Scrambled	0.42	0.26	0.16	0.37	0.46	1.46	0.14	5.50	0.13	2.15	0	0	11.05
	Egg and cheese dishes													
174	**Cauliflower cheese**	0.16	0.10	0.06	0.14	0.19	0.72	0.06	1.84	0.08	0.77	0.05	0.05	4.22
175	**Cheese pudding**	0.24	0.15	0.09	0.21	0.27	0.86	0.08	2.61	0.08	1.05	Tr	0	5.64
176	**Cheese souffle**	0.23	0.15	0.09	0.20	0.27	1.21	0.08	4.19	0.14	1.65	0.14	0.14	8.49
177	**Macaroni cheese**	0.20	0.12	0.07	0.17	0.23	0.85	0.07	2.18	0.09	0.91	0.05	0.05	4.99
178	**Pizza**, cheese and tomato	0.23	0.14	0.09	0.20	0.25	0.80	0.08	2.31	0.07	0.88	0.01	0.05	5.06
179	**Quiche Lorraine**	0.24	0.15	0.09	0.21	0.28	1.31	0.08	6.67	0.13	3.16	0.09	0.09	12.50
180	**Scotch egg**	0	0	0	0	0	0.29	0	5.09	0	2.45	0	0	7.83
181	**Welsh rarebit**	0.69	0.43	0.26	0.60	0.76	2.41	0.24	5.74	0.21	2.44	0	0	13.78

Fatty acids (g per 100 g food)

No	Food	Mono-unsaturated								Polyunsaturated							
		14:1	15:1	16:1	17:1	18:1	20:1	22:1	Total	18:2	18:3	20:4	20:5	22:6	20:1-20:5	22:5& 22:6	Total
	Eggs																
165	Whole raw	0	0	0.38	0	3.88	0	0	4.26	1.00	0	0.07	C	0.11	N	N	1.18
167	Yolk raw	0	0	1.06	0	10.86	0	0	11.92	2.81	0	0.20	C	0.30	N	N	3.31
168	Dried	0	0	1.51	0	15.42	0	0	16.93	3.99	0	0.29	C	0.43	N	N	4.71
169	Boiled	0	0	0.38	0	3.88	0	0	4.26	1.00	0	0.07	C	0.11	N	N	1.18
171	Poached	0	0	0.41	0	4.17	0	0	4.58	1.08	0	0.08	C	0.12	N	N	1.28
172	Omelette	0.05	0.02	0.43	0.04	4.37	0	0	4.91	0.94	0.05	0.06	0	0.10	N	N	1.15
173	Scrambled	0.18	0.09	0.66	0.14	6.79	0	0	7.86	1.00	0.20	0.06	0	0.09	N	N	1.35
	Egg and cheese dishes																
174	**Cauliflower cheese**	0.07	0.04	0.28	0.06	1.98	0.21	0.22	2.86	0.27	0.09	0.04	0.14	0	N	0.10	0.64
175	**Cheese pudding**	0.11	0.05	0.29	0.08	3.04	0	0	3.57	0.42	0.12	0.02	0	0.02	N	N	0.58
176	**Cheese souffle**	0.10	0.05	0.73	0.08	4.92	0.59	0.61	7.08	0.86	0.13	0.12	0.40	0.04	N	0.28	1.83
177	**Macaroni cheese**	0.09	0.04	0.32	0.07	2.34	0.23	0.24	3.33	0.33	0.11	0.03	0.16	0	N	0.11	0.74
178	**Pizza**, cheese and tomato	0.10	0.05	0.23	0.08	4.44	0	0	4.90	0.59	0.14	0	0	0	0	0	0.73
179	**Quiche Lorraine**	0.11	0.05	0.91	0.08	8.96	0.47	0.40	10.98	1.58	0.21	0.07	0.27	0.02	N	0.18	2.33
180	**Scotch egg**	0	0	0.72	0	8.65	0.08	0	9.45	1.66	0.09	0.03	0	0.05	N	N	1.83
181	**Welsh rarebit**	0.30	0.15	0.59	0.24	6.09	0	0	7.37	0.63	0.34	0	0	0	0	0	0.97

Fats & oils

Fatty acids (g per 100 g food)

No	Food	Saturated													Total
		4:0	6:0	8:0	10:0	12:0	14:0	15:0	16:0	17:0	18:0	20:0	22:0	24:0	
140	**Butter** salted	2.48	1.55	0.93	2.17	2.71	8.68	0.85	20.15	0.77	8.68	0	0	0	48.97
183	**Compound cooking fat**[a]	0	0	0	0	0.38	5.89	0	21.07	0	8.07	2.47	2.09	0	39.97
184	**Dripping** beef	0	0	0	0	0	3.03	0.57	25.46	1.14	12.30	0	0	0	42.50
185	**Lard**	0	0	0	0	0	1.51	0	25.36	0.19	14.76	0	0	0	41.82
186	**Low fat spread**[a]	0	0	0	0	2.26	1.13	0	5.33	0	1.87	0.19	0.19	0	10.97
188	**Margarine** hard, animal and vegetable oils[a]	0	0	0	0	0.23	4.49	0	15.18	0.77	6.04	1.54	1.54	0	29.79
189	hard, vegetable oils only[a]	0	0	0	0	0.08	0.93	0	21.68	0.23	5.73	0.77	0.39	0	29.81
190	soft, animal and vegetable oils[a]	0	0	0	0	0.77	3.48	0	12.16	0.70	4.10	1.32	1.94	0	24.47
191	soft, vegetable oils only[a]	0	0	0	0	1.16	1.08	0	18.35	0	4.03	0.62	0.39	0	25.63
192	polyunsaturated[a]	0	0	0	0	2.01	1.08	0	8.36	0	6.74	0.39	0.54	0	19.12
193	**Suet** block	0	0	0	0	0	3.12	0.47	26.31	1.14	25.18	0	0	0	56.22
194	shredded	0	0	0	0	0	2.74	0.41	23.04	0.99	22.05	0	0	0	49.23
196	**Coconut oil**	0	0	7.06	6.68	44.89	14.87	0	8.47	0	2.26	0.94	0	0	85.17
197	**Cottonseed oil**	0	0	0	0	0.38	0.76	0	21.97	0	2.29	0.19	0	0	25.59
198	**Maize (corn) oil**	0	0	0	0	0	0.57	0	13.37	0	2.20	0.29	0	0	16.43
199	**Olive oil**	0	0	0	0	0	0	0	11.46	0	2.20	0.38	0	0	14.04
200	**Palm oil**	0	0	0	0	0.19	1.05	0	39.63	0	4.11	0.29	0	0	45.27
201	**Peanut, groundnut, arachis oil**	0	0	0	0	0.10	0.48	0	10.22	0	2.58	1.15	3.25	1.05	18.83
202	**Rapeseed oil** high erucic acid	0	0	0	0	0	0	0	3.34	0	0.96	0.76	0.19	0.10	5.35
203	low erucic acid	0	0	0	0	0	0	0	4.30	0	1.15	0.76	0.29	0.10	6.60
204	**Safflower seed oil**	0	0	0	0	0	0	0	7.64	0	2.39	0.19	0	0	10.22
205	**Soyabean oil**	0	0	0	0	0.10	0.19	0	9.55	0	3.82	0.29	0.10	0	14.05
206	**Sunflower seed oil**	0	0	0	0	0	0.10	0	5.54	0	6.02	0.57	0.67	0.19	13.09
207	**Wheat germ oil**	0	0	0	0	0	0	0	13.08	0	0.70	0.56	0	0	14.34

[a] As these products are made from a mixture of oils and fats, the composition may vary throughout the year, depending on raw materials

Fatty acids (g per 100 g food)

No	Food	Mono-unsaturated								Polyunsaturated							
		14:1	15:1	16:1	17:1	18:1	20:1	22:1	Total	18:2	18:3	20:4	20:5	22:6	20:1-20:5	22:5-22:6	Total
140	**Butter** salted	1.08	0.54	2.09	0.85	21.54	0	0	26.10	1.08	1.16	0	0	0	0	0	2.24
183	**Compound cooking fat**[a]	0	0	6.17	0	18.51	7.59	7.88	40.15	4.75	0.47	(1.23)	(4.75)	N	N	2.85	14.05
184	**Dripping** beef	1.42	0	5.96	0.95	39.75	0	0	48.08	1.89	1.23	0.95	0	0	N	0	4.07
185	**Lard**	0	0	2.37	0	38.52	0.76	0	41.65	8.23	0.76	0	0	0	N	0	8.99
186	**Low fat spread**[a]	0	0	0.23	0	12.14	0.74	2.41	15.52	10.78	1.09	(0.04)	(0.15)	0	N	0	12.06
188	**Margarine** hard, animal and vegetable oils[a]	0	0	4.49	0	16.73	6.58	6.81	34.61	3.56	1.55	(1.08)	(4.49)	N	N	3.10	13.78
189	hard, vegetable oils only[a]	0	0	0.93	0	32.99	1.24	2.71	37.87	7.67	0.39	(0.15)	(0.77)	N	N	0.77	9.75
190	soft, animal and vegetable oils[a]	0	0	4.26	0	19.90	5.03	7.28	36.47	6.81	0.31	(1.01)	(4.18)	N	N	3.48	15.79
191	soft, vegetable oils only[a]	0	0	1.08	0	28.58	1.08	2.94	33.68	16.33	1.55	Tr	Tr	N	Tr	Tr	17.88
192	polyunsaturated[a]	0	0	0.31	0	14.56	0.46	0.54	15.87	41.58	0.54	Tr	(0.15)	0	N	Tr	60.15
193	**Suet** block	0	0.57	2.08	1.51	32.46	0	0	36.62	1.23	0	0	0	0	0	0	1.23
194	shredded	0	0.50	1.82	1.33	28.43	0	0	32.08	1.08	0	0	0	0	0	0	1.08
196	**Coconut oil**	0	0	0.38	0	6.21	0	0	6.59	1.69	0	0	0	0	0	0	1.69
197	**Cottonseed oil**	0	0	1.24	0	20.06	0	0	21.30	46.80	1.34	0	0	0	0	0	48.14
198	**Maize (corn) oil**	0	0	0.29	0	28.65	0.19	0.19	29.32	47.75	1.53	0	0	0	0	0	49.28
199	**Olive oil**	0	0	0.96	0	68.76	0	0	69.72	10.51	0.67	0	0	0	0	0	11.18
200	**Palm oil**	0	0	0.29	0	41.35	0	0	41.64	8.02	0.29	0	0	0	0	0	8.31
201	**Peanut, groundnut, arachis oil**	0	0	0	0	46.80	1.05	0	47.85	27.70	0.76	0	0	0	0	0	28.46
202	**Rapeseed oil** high erucic acid	0	0	0.19	0	23.02	9.55	31.52	64.28	14.80	10.03	0	0	0	0	0	24.83
203	low erucic acid	0	0	2.29	0	51.57	1.43	1.91	57.20	21.97	9.55	0	0	0	0	0	31.52
204	**Safflower seed oil**	0	0	0.10	0	12.42	0.10	0	12.62	71.63	0.48	0	0	0	0	0	72.11
205	**Soyabean oil**	0	0	0.19	0	23.88	0.19	0	24.26	49.66	7.07	0	0	0	0	0	56.73
206	**Sunflower seed oil**	0	0	0.10	0	31.52	0.19	0	31.81	49.66	0.29	0	0	0	0	0	49.95
207	**Wheat germ oil**	0	0	0.35	0	10.70	0.28	0	11.33	41.54	2.87	0.14	0	0	0	0	44.55

[a] As these products are made from a mixture of oils and fats, the composit on may vary throughout the year, depending on raw materials

Meat and meat products

Fatty acids (g per 100 g food)

No	Food	Saturated												Total
		4:0	6:0	8:0	10:0	12:0	14:0	15:0	16:0	17:0	18:0	20:0	22:0	
	Bacon													
208	**dressed carcase**, raw	0	0	0	0	0	0.50	0	8.50	0	4.44	0	0	13.44
210	**lean** average, raw	0	0	0	0	0	0.11	0	1.89	0	0.99	0	0	2.99
211	**fat**, average raw	0	0	0	0	0	1.21	0	20.66	0	10.78	0	0	32.65
212	cooked	0	0	0	0	0	1.09	0	18.59	0	9.70	0	0	29.38
213	**collar joint** raw, lean and fat	0	0	0	0	0	0.43	0	7.38	0	3.85	0	0	11.66
214	boiled, lean and fat	0	0	0	0	0	0.40	0	6.89	0	3.60	0	0	10.89
215	lean only	0	0	0	0	0	0.14	0	2.48	0	1.29	0	0	3.91
216	**gammon joint** raw, lean and fat	0	0	0	0	0	0.27	0	4.67	0	2.44	0	0	7.38
217	boiled, lean and fat	0	0	0	0	0	0.28	0	4.83	0	2.52	0	0	7.63
218	lean only	0	0	0	0	0	0.08	0	1.40	0	0.73	0	0	2.21
219	**gammon rashers**, grilled, lean and fat	0	0	0	0	0	0.18	0	3.12	0	1.63	0	0	4.93
220	lean only	0	0	0	0	0	0.08	0	1.33	0	0.69	0	0	2.10
221	**rashers, raw** back, lean and fat	0	0	0	0	0	0.61	0	10.52	0	5.49	0	0	16.62
222	middle, lean and fat	0	0	0	0	0	0.61	0	10.44	0	5.45	0	0	16.50
223	streaky, lean and fat	0	0	0	0	0	0.59	0	10.09	0	5.26	0	0	15.94
225	**rashers, fried** average, lean only	0	0	0	0	0	0.33	0	5.69	0	2.97	0	0	8.99
226	back, lean and fat	0	0	0	0	0	0.61	0	10.37	0	5.41	0	0	16.39
227	middle, lean and fat	0	0	0	0	0	0.63	0	10.80	0	5.64	0	0	17.07
228	streaky, lean and fat	0	0	0	0	0	0.67	0	11.44	0	5.97	0	0	18.08
230	**rashers, grilled** average, lean only	0	0	0	0	0	0.28	0	4.83	0	2.52	0	0	7.63
231	back, lean and fat	0	0	0	0	0	0.50	0	8.63	0	4.50	0	0	13.63
232	middle, lean and fat	0	0	0	0	0	0.52	0	8.96	0	4.68	0	0	14.16
233	streaky, lean and fat	0	0	0	0	0	0.54	0	9.19	0	4.80	0	0	14.53

Fatty acids (g per 100 g food)

No	Food	Mono-unsaturated								Polyunsaturated						
		14:1	15:1	16:1	17:1	18:1	20:1	22:1	Total	18:2	18:3	20:4	20:5	22:5	22:6	Total
	Bacon															
208	**dressed carcase**, raw	0	0	1.09	0	13.59	0.19	0	14.87	2.23	0.19	0	0	0	0	2.42
210	**lean** average, raw	0	0	0.24	0	3.02	0.04	0	3.30	0.50	0.04	0	0	0	0	0.54
211	**fat**, average raw	0	0	2.64	0	33.02	0.45	0	36.11	5.43	0.45	0	0	0	0	5.88
212	cooked	0	0	2.37	0	29.72	0.41	0	32.50	4.89	0.41	0	0	0	0	5.30
213	**collar joint** raw, lean and fat	0	0	0.94	0	11.80	0.16	0	12.90	1.94	0.16	0	0	0	0	2.10
214	boiled, lean and fat	0	0	0.88	0	11.02	0.15	0	12.05	1.81	0.15	0	0	0	0	1.96
215	lean only	0	0	0.32	0	3.96	0.05	0	4.33	0.65	0.05	0	0	0	0	0.70
216	**gammon joint** raw, lean and fat	0	0	0.60	0	7.47	0.10	0	8.17	1.23	0.10	0	0	0	0	1.33
217	boiled, lean and fat	0	0	0.62	0	7.72	0.11	0	8.45	1.27	0.11	0	0	0	0	1.38
218	lean only	0	0	0.18	0	2.25	0.03	0	2.46	0.37	0.03	0	0	0	0	0.40
219	**gammon rashers**, grilled, lean and fat	0	0	0.40	0	4.98	0.07	0	5.45	0.82	0.07	0	0	0	0	0.89
220	lean only	0	0	0.17	0	2.12	0.03	0	2.32	0.35	0.03	0	0	0	0	0.38
221	**rashers, raw** back, lean and fat	0	0	1.34	0	16.82	0.23	0	18.39	2.76	0.23	0	0	0	0	2.99
222	middle, lean and fat	0	0	1.33	0	16.70	0.23	0	18.26	2.74	0.23	0	0	0	0	2.97
223	streaky, lean and fat	0	0	1.29	0	16.12	0.22	0	17.63	2.65	0.22	0	0	0	0	2.87
225	**rashers, fried** average, lean only	0	0	0.73	0	9.10	0.12	0	9.95	1.50	0.12	0	0	0	0	1.62
226	back, lean and fat	0	0	1.32	0	16.57	0.23	0	18.12	2.72	0.23	0	0	0	0	2.95
227	middle, lean and fat	0	0	1.38	0	17.27	0.24	0	18.89	2.84	0.24	0	0	0	0	3.08
228	streaky, lean and fat	0	0	1.46	0	18.29	0.25	0	20.00	3.01	0.25	0	0	0	0	3.26
230	**rashers, grilled** average, lean only	0	0	0.62	0	7.72	0.11	0	8.45	1.27	0.11	0	0	0	0	1.38
231	back, lean and fat	0	0	1.10	0	13.80	0.19	0	15.09	2.27	0.19	0	0	0	0	2.46
232	middle, lean and fat	0	0	1.14	0	14.33	0.20	0	15.67	2.36	0.20	0	0	0	0	2.56
233	streaky, lean and fat	0	0	1.17	0	14.70	0.20	0	16.07	2.42	0.20	0	0	0	0	2.62

Fatty acids (g per 100 g food)

No	Food	Saturated												Total
		4:0	6:0	8:0	10:0	12:0	14:0	15:0	16:0	17:0	18:0	20:0	22:0	
	Beef													
235	**dressed carcase**, raw	0	0	0	0	0	0.73	0.14	6.11	0.27	2.95	0	0	10.20
237	**lean** average, raw	0	0	0	0	0	0.14	0.03	1.16	0.05	0.56	0	0	1.94
240	**fat** average raw	0	0	0	0	0	2.00	0.38	16.83	0.75	8.13	0	0	28.09
241	cooked	0	0	0	0	0	1.88	0.35	15.80	0.70	7.63	0	0	26.36
242	**brisket** raw, lean and fat	0	0	0	0	0	0.61	0.12	5.16	0.23	2.49	0	0	8.61
243	boiled, lean and fat	0	0	0	0	0	0.72	0.13	6.01	0.27	2.91	0	0	10.04
244	**forerib** raw, lean and fat	0	0	0	0	0	0.75	0.14	6.31	0.28	3.05	0	0	10.53
245	roast, lean and fat	0	0	0	0	0	0.86	0.16	7.24	0.32	3.50	0	0	12.08
246	lean only	0	0	0	0	0	0.38	0.07	3.17	0.14	1.53	0	0	5.29
247	**mince** raw	0	0	0	0	0	0.48	0.09	4.07	0.18	1.97	0	0	6.79
248	stewed	0	0	0	0	0	0.45	0.09	3.82	0.17	1.85	0	0	6.38
249	**rump steak** raw, lean and fat	0	0	0	0	0	0.40	0.08	3.40	0.15	1.64	0	0	5.67
250	fried, lean and fat	0	0	0	0	0	0.44	0.08	3.67	0.16	1.77	0	0	6.12
251	lean only	0	0	0	0	0	0.22	0.04	1.86	0.08	0.90	0	0	3.10
252	grilled, lean and fat	0	0	0	0	0	0.36	0.07	3.04	0.14	1.47	0	0	5.08
253	lean only	0	0	0	0	0	0.18	0.03	1.51	0.07	0.73	0	0	2.52
254	**silverside** salted, boiled, lean and fat	0	0	0	0	0	0.42	0.08	3.57	0.16	1.73	0	0	5.96
255	lean only	0	0	0	0	0	0.15	0.03	1.23	0.05	0.60	0	0	2.06
256	**sirloin** raw, lean and fat	0	0	0	0	0	0.68	0.13	5.73	0.26	2.77	0	0	9.57
257	roast, lean and fat	0	0	0	0	0	0.63	0.12	5.31	0.24	2.56	0	0	8.86
258	lean only	0	0	0	0	0	0.27	0.05	2.29	0.10	1.11	0	0	3.82
259	**stewing steak** raw, lean and fat	0	0	0	0	0	0.32	0.06	2.67	0.12	1.29	0	0	4.46
260	stewed, lean and fat	0	0	0	0	0	0.33	0.06	2.77	0.12	1.34	0	0	4.62
261	**topside** raw, lean and fat	0	0	0	0	0	0.34	0.06	2.82	0.13	1.36	0	0	4.71
262	roast, lean and fat	0	0	0	0	0	0.36	0.07	3.02	0.13	1.46	0	0	5.04
263	lean only	0	0	0	0	0	0.13	0.02	1.11	0.05	0.53	0	0	1.84

Fatty acids (g per 100 g food)

No	Food	Mono-unsaturated								Polyunsaturated							
		14:1	15:1	16:1	17:1	18:1	20:1	22:1	Total	18:2	18:3	20:3	20:4	20:5	22:5	22:6	Total
	Beef																
235	**dressed carcase**, raw	0.34	0	1.43	0.23	9.54	0	0	11.54	0.45	0.30	0	0.23	0	0	0	0.98
237	**lean** average, raw	0.06	0	0.27	0.04	1.81	0	0	2.18	0.09	0.06	0	0.04	0	0	0	0.19
240	**fat** average raw	0.94	0	3.94	0.63	26.27	0	0	31.78	1.25	0.81	0	0.63	0	0	0	2.69
241	cooked	0.88	0	3.70	0.59	24.66	0	0	29.83	1.17	0.76	0	0.59	0	0	0	2.52
242	**brisket** raw, lean and fat	0.29	0	1.21	0.19	8.05	0	0	9.74	0.38	0.25	0	0.19	0	0	0	0.82
243	boiled, lean and fat	0.34	0	1.41	0.22	9.39	0	0	1.36	0.45	0.29	0	0.22	0	0	0	0.96
244	**forerib** raw, lean and fat	0.35	0	1.48	0.23	9.86	0	0	1.92	0.47	0.31	0	0.23	0	0	0	1.01
245	roast, lean and fat	0.40	0	1.70	0.27	11.31	0	0	3.68	0.54	0.35	0	0.27	0	0	0	1.16
246	lean only	0.18	0	0.74	0.12	4.95	0	0	5.99	0.24	0.15	0	0.12	0	0	0	0.51
247	**mince** raw	0.23	0	0.95	0.15	6.36	0	0	7.69	0.30	0.20	0	0.15	0	0	0	0.65
248	stewed	0.21	0	0.90	0.14	5.97	0	0	7.22	0.28	0.18	0	0.14	0	0	0	0.60
249	**rump steak** raw, lean and fat	0.19	0	0.80	0.13	5.30	0	0	6.42	0.25	0.16	0	0.13	0	0	0	0.54
250	fried, lean and fat	0.20	0	0.86	0.14	5.73	0	0	6.93	0.27	0.18	0	0.14	0	0	0	0.59
251	lean only	0.10	0	0.44	0.07	2.91	0	0	3.52	0.14	0.09	0	0.07	0	0	0	0.30
252	grilled, lean and fat	0.17	0	0.71	0.11	4.75	0	0	5.74	0.23	0.15	0	0.11	0	0	0	0.49
253	lean only	0.08	0	0.35	0.06	2.36	0	0	2.85	0.11	0.07	0	0.06	0	0	0	0.24
254	**silverside** salted, boiled, lean and fat	0.20	0	0.84	0.13	5.58	0	0	6.75	0.27	0.17	0	0.13	0	0	0	0.57
255	lean only	0.07	0	0.29	0.05	1.92	0	0	2.33	0.09	0.06	0	0.05	0	0	0	0.20
256	**sirloin** raw, lean and fat	0.32	0	1.34	0.21	8.95	0	0	10.82	0.43	0.28	0	0.21	0	0	0	0.92
257	roast, lean and fat	0.30	0	1.24	0.20	8.29	0	0	10.03	0.39	0.26	0	0.20	0	0	0	0.85
258	lean only	0.13	0	0.54	0.09	3.57	0	0	4.33	0.17	0.11	0	0.09	0	0	0	0.37
259	**stewing steak** raw, lean and fat	0.15	0	0.62	0.10	4.16	0	0	5.03	0.20	0.13	0	0.10	0	0	0	0.43
260	stewed, lean and fat	0.15	0	0.65	0.10	4.32	0	0	5.22	0.21	0.13	0	0.10	0	0	0	0.44
261	**topside** raw, lean and fat	0.16	0	0.66	0.10	4.40	0	0	5.32	0.21	0.14	0	0.10	0	0	0	0.45
262	roast, lean and fat	0.17	0	0.71	0.11	4.71	0	0	5.70	0.22	0.15	0	0.11	0	0	0	0.48
263	lean only	0.06	0	0.26	0.04	1.73	0	0	2.09	0.08	0.05	0	0.04	0	0	0	0.17

Meat *continued*

Fatty acids (g per 100 g food)

No	Food	Saturated												Total
		4:0	6:0	8:0	10:0	12:0	14:0	15:0	16:0	17:0	18:0	20:0	22:0	
	Lamb													
264	**dressed carcase**, raw	0	0	0	0	0	1.54	0.17	6.90	0.29	5.96	0	0	14.86
266	**lean** average, raw	0	0	0	0	0	0.44	0.05	1.99	0.08	1.72	0	0	4.28
269	**fat** average, raw	0	0	0	0	0	3.63	0.40	16.25	0.67	14.03	0	0	34.98
270	cooked	0	0	0	0	0	3.20	0.36	14.35	0.59	12.39	0	0	30.89
271	**breast** raw, lean and fat	0	0	0	0	0	1.75	0.19	7.83	0.32	6.76	0	0	16.85
272	roast, lean and fat	0	0	0	0	0	1.87	0.21	8.39	0.35	7.25	0	0	18.07
273	lean only	0	0	0	0	0	0.84	0.09	3.76	0.16	3.24	0	0	8.09
274	**chops, loin** raw, lean and fat	0	0	0	0	0	1.79	0.20	8.01	0.33	6.92	0	0	17.25
275	grilled, lean and fat	0	0	0	0	0	1.46	0.16	6.56	0.27	5.67	0	0	14.12
276	lean and fat (weighed with bone)	0	0	0	0	0	1.14	0.13	5.11	0.21	4.42	0	0	11.01
277	lean only	0	0	0	0	0	0.62	0.07	2.78	0.12	2.40	0	0	5.99
278	lean only (weighed with fat and bone)	0	0	0	0	0	0.34	0.04	1.54	0.06	1.33	0	0	3.31
279	**cutlets** raw, lean and fat	0	0	0	0	0	1.83	0.20	8.21	0.34	7.09	0	0	17.67
280	grilled, lean and fat	0	0	0	0	0	1.56	0.17	6.99	0.29	6.04	0	0	15.05
281	lean and fat (weighed with bone)	0	0	0	0	0	1.03	0.11	4.62	0.19	3.99	0	0	9.94
282	lean only	0	0	0	0	0	0.62	0.07	2.78	0.12	2.40	0	0	5.99
283	lean only (weighed with fat and bone)	0	0	0	0	0	0.27	0.03	1.22	0.05	1.06	0	0	2.63
284	**leg** raw, lean and fat	0	0	0	0	0	0.94	0.10	4.23	0.17	3.65	0	0	9.09
285	roast, lean and fat	0	0	0	0	0	0.90	0.10	4.05	0.17	3.50	0	0	8.72
286	lean only	0	0	0	0	0	0.41	0.05	1.83	0.08	1.58	0	0	3.95
287	**scrag and neck** raw, lean and fat	0	0	0	0	0	1.42	0.16	6.38	0.26	5.51	0	0	13.73
288	stewed, lean and fat	0	0	0	0	0	1.07	0.12	4.77	0.20	4.12	0	0	10.28
289	lean only	0	0	0	0	0	0.79	0.09	3.55	0.15	3.07	0	0	7.65
290	lean only (weighed with fat and bone)	0	0	0	0	0	0.40	0.04	1.81	0.07	1.56	0	0	3.88

No	Food	Mono-unsaturated								Polyunsaturated							
		14:1	15:1	16:1	17:1	18:1	20:1	22:1	Total	18:2	18:3	20:3	20:4	20:5	22:5	22:6	Total
	Lamb																
264	**dressed carcase,** raw	0	0	0.37	0.29	10.89	0	0	11.55	0.71	0.71	0	0	0	0	0	1.42
266	**lean** average, raw	0	0	0.11	0.08	3.14	0	0	3.33	0.21	0.21	0	0	0	0	0	0.42
269	**fat** average, raw	0	0	0.87	0.67	25.64	0	0	27.18	1.68	1.68	0	0	0	0	0	3.36
270	cooked	0	0	0.77	0.59	22.64	0	0	24.00	1.48	1.48	0	0	0	0	0	2.96
271	**breast** raw, lean and fat	0	0	0.42	0.32	12.36	0	0	13.10	0.81	0.81	0	0	0	0	0	1.62
272	roast, lean and fat	0	0	0.45	0.35	13.25	0	0	14.05	0.87	0.87	0	0	0	0	0	1.74
273	lean only	0	0	0.20	0.16	5.93	0	0	6.29	0.39	0.39	0	0	0	0	0	0.78
274	**chops, loin** raw, lean and fat	0	0	0.43	0.33	12.64	0	0	13.40	0.83	0.83	0	0	0	0	0	1.66
275	grilled, lean and fat	0	0	0.35	0.27	10.36	0	0	10.98	0.68	0.68	0	0	0	0	0	1.36
276	lean and fat (weighed with bone)	0	0	0.27	0.21	8.07	0	0	8.55	0.53	0.53	0	0	0	0	0	1.06
277	lean only	0	0	0.15	0.12	4.39	0	0	4.66	0.29	0.29	0	0	0	0	0	0.58
278	lean only (weighed with fat and bone)	0	0	0.08	0.06	2.43	0	0	2.57	0.16	0.16	0	0	0	0	0	0.32
279	**cutlets** raw, lean and fat	0	0	0.44	0.34	12.97	0	0	13.75	0.85	0.85	0	0	0	0	0	1.70
280	grilled, lean and fat	0	0	0.38	0.29	11.04	0	0	11.71	0.72	0.72	0	0	0	0	0	1.44
281	lean and fat (weighed with bone)	0	0	0.25	0.19	7.29	0	0	7.73	0.48	0.48	0	0	0	0	0	0.96
282	lean only	0	0	0.15	0.12	4.39	0	0	4.66	0.29	0.29	0	0	0	0	0	0.58
283	lean only (weighed with fat and bone)	0	0	0.07	0.05	1.93	0	0	2.05	0.13	0.13	0	0	0	0	0	0.26
284	**leg** raw, lean and fat	0	0	0.23	0.17	6.68	0	0	7.08	0.44	0.44	0	0	0	0	0	0.88
285	roast, lean and fat	0	0	0.22	0.17	6.39	0	0	6.78	0.42	0.42	0	0	0	0	0	0.84
286	lean only	0	0	0.10	0.08	2.89	0	0	3.07	0.19	0.19	0	0	0	0	0	0.38
287	**scrag and neck** raw, lean and fat	0	0	0.34	0.26	10.07	0	0	10.67	0.66	0.66	0	0	0	0	0	1.32
288	stewed, lean and fat	0	0	0.26	0.20	7.54	0	0	8.00	0.49	0.49	0	0	0	0	0	0.98
289	lean only	0	0	0.19	0.15	5.61	0	0	5.95	0.37	0.37	0	0	0	0	0	0.74
290	lean only (weighed with fat and bone)	0	0	0.10	0.07	2.86	0	0	3.03	0.19	0.19	0	0	0	0	0	0.38

Meat *continued*

Fatty acids (g per 100 g food)

No	Food	Saturated 4:0	6:0	8:0	10:0	12:0	14:0	15:0	16:0	17:0	18:0	20:0	22:0	Total
	Lamb contd													
291	**shoulder** raw, lean and fat	0	0	0	0	0	1.41	0.16	6.34	0.26	5.47	0	0	13.64
292	roast, lean and fat	0	0	0	0	0	1.33	0.15	5.95	0.25	5.14	0	0	12.82
293	lean only	0	0	0	0	0	0.57	0.06	2.53	0.10	2.19	0	0	5.45
	Pork													
294	**dressed carcase** raw	0	0	0	0	0	0.47	0	7.96	0	4.05	0	0	12.48
296	**lean** average, raw	0	0	0	0	0	0.11	0	1.79	0	0.91	0	0	2.81
299	**fat** average, raw	0	0	0	0	0	1.06	0	18.03	0	9.18	0	0	28.27
300	cooked	0	0	0	0	0	0.93	0	15.71	0	8.00	0	0	24.64
	belly, rashers													
301	raw, lean and fat	0	0	0	0	0	0.53	0	8.97	0	4.57	0	0	14.07
302	grilled, lean and fat	0	0	0	0	0	0.52	0	8.79	0	4.48	0	0	13.79
	chops, loin raw,													
303	lean and fat	0	0	0	0	0	0.44	0	7.45	0	3.79	0	0	11.68
304	grilled, lean and fat	0	0	0	0	0	0.36	0	6.11	0	3.11	0	0	9.58
305	lean and fat (weighed with bone)	0	0	0	0	0	0.28	0	4.75	0	2.42	0	0	7.45
306	lean only	0	0	0	0	0	0.16	0	2.70	0	1.38	0	0	4.24
307	lean only (weighed with fat and bone)	0	0	0	0	0	0.09	0	1.59	0	0.81	0	0	2.49
308	**leg** raw, lean and fat	0	0	0	0	0	0.34	0	5.68	0	2.89	0	0	8.91
309	roast, lean and fat	0	0	0	0	0	0.30	0	5.00	0	2.55	0	0	7.85
310	lean only	0	0	0	0	0	0.10	0	1.74	0	0.89	0	0	2.73
	Veal													
311	**cutlet** fried	0	0	0	0	0	0.24	0.05	2.04	0.09	0.98	0	0	3.40
312	**fillet** raw	0	0	0	0	0	0.08	0.02	0.68	0.03	0.33	0	0	1.14
313	roast	0	0	0	0	0	0.34	0.06	2.89	0.13	1.40	0	0	4.82

Fatty acids (g per 100 g food)

No	Food	Mono-unsaturated								Polyunsaturated							
		14:1	15:1	16:1	17:1	18:1	20:1	22:1	Total	18:2	18:3	20:3	20:4	20:5	22:5	22:6	Total
	Lamb contd																
	shoulder raw,																
291	lean and fat	0	0	0.34	0.26	10.00	0	0	10.60	0.65	0.65	0	0	0	0	0	1.30
292	roast, lean and fat	0	0	0.32	0.25	9.39	0	0	9.96	0.61	0.61	0	0	0	0	0	1.22
293	lean only	0	0	0.14	0.10	4.00	0	0	4.24	0.26	0.26	0	0	0	0	0	0.52
	Pork																
294	**dressed carcase** raw	0	0	1.00	0	12.86	0.21	0	14.07	2.17	0.26	0	0	0	0	0	2.43
296	**lean** average, raw	0	0	0.22	0	2.90	0.05	0	3.17	0.49	0.06	0	0	0	0	0	0.55
299	**fat** average, raw	0	0	2.26	0	29.15	0.47	0	31.88	4.92	0.60	0	0	0	0	0	5.52
300	cooked	0	0	1.97	0	25.39	0.41	0	27.77	4.29	0.52	0	0	0	0	0	4.81
	belly, rashers																
301	raw, lean and fat	0	0	1.12	0	14.49	0.23	0	15.84	2.45	0.30	0	0	0	0	0	2.75
302	grilled, lean and fat	0	0	1.10	0	14.21	0.23	0	15.54	2.40	0.29	0	0	0	0	0	2.69
303	**chops, loin** raw, lean and fat	0	0	0.93	0	12.04	0.19	0	13.16	2.03	0.25	0	0	0	0	0	2.28
304	grilled, lean and fat	0	0	0.77	0	9.88	0.16	0	10.81	1.67	0.20	0	0	0	0	0	1.87
305	lean and fat (weighed with bone)	0	0	0.60	0	7.67	0.12	0	8.39	1.30	0.16	0	0	0	0	0	1.46
306	lean only	0	0	0.34	0	4.37	0.07	0	4.78	0.74	0.09	0	0	0	0	0	0.83
307	lean only (weighed with fat and bone)	0	0	0.20	0	2.57	0.04	0	2.81	0.43	0.05	0	0	0	0	0	0.48
308	**leg** raw, lean and fat	0	0	0.71	0	9.18	0.15	0	10.04	1.55	0.19	0	0	0	0	0	1.74
309	roast, lean and fat	0	0	0.63	0	8.08	0.13	0	8.84	1.37	0.17	0	0	0	0	0	1.54
310	lean only	0	0	0.22	0	2.82	0.05	0	3.05	0.48	0.06	0	0	0	0	0	0.54
	Veal																
311	**cutlet** fried	0.11	0	0.48	0.08	3.18	0	0	3.85	0.15	0.10	0	0.08	0	0	0	0.33
312	**fillet** raw	0.04	0	0.16	0.03	1.06	0	0	1.29	0.05	0.03	0	0.03	0	0	0	0.11
313	roast	0.16	0	0.68	0.11	4.52	0	0	5.47	0.22	0.14	0	0.11	0	0	0	0.47

Meat *continued*

Fatty acids (g per 100 g food)

No	Food	Saturated												Total
		4:0	6:0	8:0	10:0	12:0	14:0	15:0	16:0	17:0	18:0	20:0	22:0	
	Poultry and game													
314	**Chicken** raw, meat only	0	0	0	0	0	0.05	0	1.08	0	0.29	0	0	1.42
315	meat and skin	0	0	0	0	0	0.22	0	4.47	0	1.19	0	0	5.88
316	light meat	0	0	0	0	0	0.04	0	0.81	0	0.21	0	0	1.06
317	dark meat	0	0	0	0	0	0.07	0	1.39	0	0.37	0	0	1.83
318	boiled, meat only	0	0	0	0	0	0.09	0	1.84	0	0.49	0	0	2.42
319	light meat	0	0	0	0	0	0.06	0	1.24	0	0.33	0	0	1.63
320	dark meat	0	0	0	0	0	0.12	0	2.50	0	0.66	0	0	3.28
321	roast, meat only	0	0	0	0	0	0.07	0	1.36	0	0.36	0	0	1.79
322	meat and skin	0	0	0	0	0	0.17	0	3.53	0	0.94	0	0	4.64
323	light meat	0	0	0	0	0	0.05	0	1.01	0	0.27	0	0	1.33
324	dark meat	0	0	0	0	0	0.08	0	1.74	0	0.46	0	0	2.28
325	wing quarter (weighed with bone)	0	0	0	0	0	0.03	0	0.68	0	0.18	0	0	0.89
326	leg quarter (weighed with bone)	0	0	0	0	0	0.04	0	0.86	0	0.23	0	0	1.13
327	**Duck** raw, meat only	0	0	0	0	0	0.03	0	1.03	0	0.25	0	0	1.31
328	meat, fat and skin	0	0	0	0	0	0.24	0	9.20	0	2.22	0	0	11.66
329	roast, meat only	0	0	0	0	0	0.05	0	2.09	0	0.50	0	0	2.64
330	meat, fat and skin	0	0	0	0	0	0.16	0	6.25	0	1.51	0	0	7.92
332	**Grouse** roast	0	0	0	0	0	0.03	Tr	0.84	0.08	0.29	0	0	1.24
333	roast (weighed with bone)	0	0	0	0	0	0.02	Tr	0.55	0.05	0.19	0	0	0.81
334	**Partridge** roast	0	0	0	0	0	0.06	Tr	1.43	0.12	0.26	0	0	1.87
335	roast (weighed with bone)	0	0	0	0	0	0.04	Tr	0.85	0.07	0.15	0	0	1.11

Fatty acids (g per 100 g food)

No	Food	Mono-unsaturated								Polyunsaturated							
		14:1	15:1	16:1	17:1	18:1	20:1	22:1	Total	18:2	18:3	20:3	20:4	20:5	22:5	22:6	Total
	Poultry and game																
314	**Chicken** raw, meat only	0	0	0.29	0	1.62	0.02	0	1.93	0.55	0.03	0	0.03	0	0	0.04	0.65
315	meat and skin	0	0	1.20	0	6.66	0.10	0	7.96	2.26	0.12	0	0.12	0	0	0.17	2.67
316	light meat	0	0	0.22	0	1.20	0.02	0	1.44	0.41	0.02	0	0.02	0	0	0.03	0.48
317	dark meat	0	0	0.37	0	2.07	0.03	0	2.47	0.70	0.04	0	0.04	0	0	0.05	0.83
318	boiled, meat only	0	0	0.50	0	2.75	0.04	0	3.29	0.93	0.05	0	0.05	0	0	0.07	1.10
319	light meat	0	0	0.33	0	1.84	0.03	0	2.20	0.63	0.03	0	0.03	0	0	0.05	0.74
320	dark meat	0	0	0.67	0	3.72	0.06	0	4.45	1.26	0.07	0	0.07	0	0	0.09	1.49
321	roast, meat only	0	0	0.37	0	2.03	0.03	0	2.43	0.69	0.04	0	0.04	0	0	0.05	0.82
322	meat and skin	0	0	0.95	0	5.27	0.08	0	6.30	1.79	0.09	0	0.09	0	0	0.13	2.10
323	light meat	0	0	0.27	0	1.50	0.02	0	1.79	0.51	0.03	0	0.03	0	0	0.04	0.61
324	dark meat	0	0	0.47	0	2.60	0.04	0	3.11	0.88	0.05	0	0.05	0	0	0.07	1.05
325	wing quarter (weighed with bone)	0	0	0.18	0	1.02	0.02	0	1.22	0.34	0.02	0	0.02	0	0	0.03	0.41
326	eg quarter (weighed with bone)	0	0	0.23	0	1.28	0.02	0	1.53	0.43	0.02	0	0.02	0	0	0.03	0.50
327	**Duck** raw, meat only	0	0	0.20	0	2.40	0	0	2.60	0.55	0.03	0	0	0	0	0	0.58
328	meat, fat and skin	0	0	1.78	0	21.31	0	0	23.09	4.88	0.24	0	0	0	0	0	5.12
329	roast, meat only	0	0	0.40	0	4.84	0	0	5.24	1.11	0.05	0	0	0	0	0	1.16
330	meat, fat and skin	0	0	1.21	0	14.47	0	0	15.68	3.32	0.16	0	0	0	0	0	3.48
332	**Grouse** roast	0	0	0.10	0.02	0.54	Tr	0	0.66	1.60	1.52	0	0	0	0	0	3.12
333	roast (weighed with bone)	0	0	0.06	Tr	0.35	Tr	0	0.41	1.06	1.00	0	0	0	0	0	2.06
334	**Partridge** roast	0	0	0.52	0.12	2.71	Tr	0	3.35	1.05	0.65	0	0	0	0	0	1.70
335	roast (weighed with bone)	0	0	0.31	0.07	1.62	Tr	0	2.00	0.63	0.39	0	0	0	0	0	1.02

Meat *continued*

Fatty acids (g per 100 g food)

Poultry and game *contd*

No	Food	Saturated												Total
		4:0	6:0	8:0	10:0	12:0	14:0	15:0	16:0	17:0	18:0	20:0	22:0	
336	**Pheasant** roast	0	0	0	0	0	0.09	Tr	2.47	Tr	0.52	0	0	3.08
337	roast (weighed with bone)	0	0	0	0	0	0.06	Tr	1.57	Tr	0.33	0	0	1.96
340	**Turkey** raw, meat only	0	0	0	0	0	0.02	0	0.52	0.01	0.21	0	0	0.76
341	meat and skin	0	0	0	0	0	0.07	0	1.63	0.03	0.65	0	0	2.38
342	light meat	0	0	0	0	0	0.01	0	0.26	Tr	0.10	0	0	0.37
343	dark meat	0	0	0	0	0	0.03	0	0.85	0.02	0.34	0	0	1.24
344	roast, meat only	0	0	0	0	0	0.03	0	0.64	0.01	0.26	0	0	0.94
345	meat and skin	0	0	0	0	0	0.06	0	1.54	0.03	0.61	0	0	2.24
346	light meat	0	0	0	0	0	0.01	0	0.33	Tr	0.13	0	0	0.47
347	dark meat	0	0	0	0	0	0.04	0	0.97	0.02	0.39	0	0	1.42
348	**Hare** stewed	0	0	0	0	0	0.20	0.05	2.27	0.06	0.70	0	0	3.28
349	stewed (weighed with bone)	0	0	0	0	0	0.14	0.04	1.64	0.04	0.50	0	0	2.36
350	**Rabbit** raw	0	0	0	0	0	0.10	0.03	1.13	0.03	0.35	0	0	1.64
351	stewed	0	0	0	0	0	0.19	0.05	2.18	0.06	0.67	0	0	3.15
352	stewed (weighed with bone)	0	0	0	0	0	0.10	0.03	1.11	0.03	0.34	0	0	1.61

Meat *continued*

Fatty acids (g per 100 g food)

No	Food	Mono-unsaturated								Polyunsaturated							
		14:1	15:1	16:1	17:1	18:1	20:1	22:1	Total	18:2	18:3	20:3	20:4	20:5	22:5	22:6	Total
	Poultry and game *contd*																
336	**Pheasant** roast	0	0	1.00	Tr	3.55	Tr	0	4.55	0.54	0.59	0	0	0	0	0	1.13
337	roast (weighed with bone)	0	0	0.64	Tr	2.25	Tr	0	2.89	0.34	0.37	0	0.10	0.03	0.04	0.10	0.71
340	**Turkey** raw, meat only	0	0	0.10	0	0.45	Tr	0	0.55	0.42	0.02	0	0.33	0.10	0.13	0.33	0.71
341	meat and skin	0	0	0.33	0	1.40	0.03	0	1.76	1.30	0.07	0	0.05	0.02	0.02	0.05	2.26
342	light meat	0	0	0.05	0	0.22	Tr	0	0.27	0.21	0.01	0	0.17	0.05	0.07	0.17	0.36
343	dark meat	0	0	0.17	0	0.73	0.01	0	0.91	0.68	0.03	0	0.17	0.05	0.07	0.17	1.17
344	roast, meat only	0	0	0.13	0	0.55	0.01	0	0.69	0.51	0.03	0	0.13	0.04	0.05	0.13	0.89
345	meat and skin	0	0	0.31	0	1.32	0.02	0	1.65	1.23	0.06	0	0.31	0.09	0.12	0.31	2.12
346	light meat	0	0	0.07	0	0.28	Tr	0	0.35	0.26	0.01	0	0.07	0.02	0.03	0.07	0.46
347	dark meat	0	0	0.19	0	0.83	0.02	0	1.04	0.77	0.04	0	0.19	0.06	0.08	0.19	1.33
348	**Hare** stewed	0	0	0.16	0	1.41	0	0	1.57	1.58	0.75	0	0.14	0	0.10	0	2.57
349	stewed (weighed with bone)	0	0	0.12	0	1.02	0	0	1.14	1.15	0.54	0	0.10	0	0.07	0	1.86
350	**Rabbit** raw	0	0	0.08	0	0.71	0	0	0.79	0.79	0.37	0	0.07	0	0.05	0	1.28
351	stewed	0	0	0.15	0	1.36	0	0	1.51	1.52	0.72	0	0.14	0	0.09	0	2.47
352	stewed (weighed with bone)	0	0	0.08	0	0.69	0	0	0.77	0.77	0.36	0	0.07	0	0.05	0	1.25

Meat *continued*

Fatty acids (g per 100 g food)

No	Food	Saturated												Total
		4:0	6:0	8:0	10:0	12:0	14:0	15:0	16:0	17:0	18:0	20:0	22:0	
	Offal													
356	**Brain, lamb** boiled	0	0	0	0	0	0.04	0.02	1.06	0.02	0.89	0	0	2.03
358	**Heart, lamb** raw	0	0	0	0	0	0.15	0.02	0.87	0.05	1.07	0	0	2.16
359	**sheep** roast	0	0	0	0	0	0.38	0.06	2.28	0.13	2.81	0	0	5.66
360	**ox** raw	0	0	0	0	0	0.09	0.02	0.78	0.04	0.83	0	0	1.76
361	stewed	0	0	0	0	0	0.15	0.04	1.28	0.06	1.36	0	0	2.89
364	**Kidney, lamb** raw	0	0	0	0	0	0.05	0	0.40	0.02	0.45	0	0	0.92
366	**ox** raw	0	0	0	0	0	0.05	0.01	0.49	0.02	0.52	0	0	1.09
367	stewed	0	0	0	0	0	0.16	0.04	1.44	0.06	1.55	0	0	3.25
368	**pig** raw	0	0	0	0	0	0.02	0	0.50	0	0.36	0	0	0.88
369	stewed	0	0	0	0	0	0.05	0	1.13	0	0.81	0	0	1.99
371	**Liver, calf** raw	0	0	0	0	0	0.04	0	0.89	0.03	1.26	0	0	2.22
373	**chicken** raw	0	0	0	0	0	0.02	0	1.15	0	0.79	0	0	1.96
375	**lamb** raw	0	0	0	0	0	0.10	0.04	1.56	0.08	1.40	0	0	3.18
377	**ox** raw	0	0	0	0	0	0.05	0.05	0.99	0.03	1.74	0	0	2.86
378	stewed	0	0	0	0	0	0.06	0.06	1.21	0.04	2.12	0	0	3.49

No	Food	Mono-unsaturated								Polyunsaturated							
		14:1	15:1	16:1	17:1	18:1	20:1	22:1	Total	18:2	18:3	20:3	20:4	20:5	22:5	22:6	Total
	Offal																
356	**Brain, lamb** boiled[a]	0	0	0.07	0.09	1.40	0.16	0.03	1.75	0.02	0	0.07	0.21	0.03	0.17	0.47	1.01
358	**Heart, lamb** raw	0	0	0.09	0.11	1.46	0	0	1.66	0.32	0.12	0	0.09	0	0	0	0.53
359	**sheep** roast	0	0	0.24	0.28	3.84	0	0	4.36	0.85	0.31	0	0.24	0	0	0	1.40
360	**ox** raw	0	0.02	0.05	0.05	0.83	0	0	0.95	0.07	0.01	0	0.02	0	0	0	0.10
361	stewed	0	0.03	0.09	0.08	1.36	0	0	1.56	0.12	0.02	0	0.03	0	0	0	0.17
364	**Kidney, lamb** raw	0	0	0.04	0.03	0.57	0	0	0.64	0.16	0.08	0.01	0.14	0	0	0	0.39
366	**ox** raw	0	0.01	0.04	0.03	0.60	0	0	0.68	0.09	Tr	0	0.05	0	0	0	0.14
367	stewed	0	0.03	0.12	0.08	1.78	0	0	2.01	0.28	0.03	0	0.15	0	0	0	0.46
368	**pig** raw	0	0	0.04	0	0.65	0.01	0	0.70	0.24	0.01	0.01	0.14	0	0	0	0.40
369	stewed	0	0	0.09	0	1.47	0.02	0	1.58	0.53	0.02	0.03	0.31	0	0	0	0.89
371	**Liver, calf** raw	0	0	0.10	0.04	1.13	0	0	1.27	0.81	0.08	0.11	0.49	0.02	0.22	0.14	1.87
373	**chicken** raw	0	0	0.15	0	1.23	0	0	1.38	0.69	0.03	0.03	0.26	0	0.04	0.22	1.27
375	**lamb** raw	0	0.04	0.27	0.12	2.27	0	0	2.70	0.38	0.29	0.05	0.39	0	0.23	0.18	1.52
377	**ox** raw	0	0.05	0.08	0.07	1.05	0	0	1.25	0.43	0.14	0.27	0.37	0.04	0.32	0.07	1.64
378	stewed	0	0.06	0.10	0.08	1.28	0	0	1.52	0.52	0.18	0.32	0.45	0.05	0.39	0.08	1.99

[a] Also contains 0.04 mg of 22:4

Fatty acids (g per 100 g food)

No	Food	Saturated													Total
		4:0	6:0	8:0	10:0	12:0	14:0	15:0	16:0	17:0	18:0	20:0	22:0		
	Offal *contd*														
379	**Liver, pig** raw	0	0	0	0	0	0	0	0.89	0.03	1.18	0	0		2.10
380	stewed	0	0	0	0	0	0	0	1.06	0.03	1.40	0	0		2.49
381	**Oxtail** raw	0	0	0	0	0	0.30	0.06	2.54	0.11	1.23	0	0		4.24
382	stewed	0	0	0	0	0	0.40	0.08	3.37	0.15	1.63	0	0		5.63
383	stewed (weighed with fat and bones)	0	0	0	0	0	0.15	0.03	1.28	0.06	0.62	0	0		2.14
384	**Sweetbread, lamb**, raw	0	0	0	0	0.04	0.29	0.04	1.27	0.06	1.31	0	0		3.01
387	**Tongue, lamb**, raw	0	0	0	0	0	0.32	0.06	2.30	0.12	1.97	0	0		4.77
388	sheep, stewed	0	0	0	0	0	0.52	0.10	3.78	0.19	3.24	0	0		7.83
391	**Tripe** dressed	0	0	0	0	0	0.06	0.02	0.47	0.03	0.61	0	0		1.19
392	stewed	0	0	0	0	0	0.10	0.03	0.84	0.05	1.10	0	0		2.12

No	Food	Mono-unsaturated								Polyunsaturated							
		14:1	15:1	16:1	17:1	18:1	20:1	22:1	Total	18:2	18:3	20:3	20:4	20:5	22:5	22:6	Total
	Offal contd																
379	**Liver, pig** raw	0	0	0.09	0	0.97	0	0	1.06	0.74	0.03	0.07	0.72	0	0.12	0.17	1.85
380	stewed	0	0	0.10	0	1.15	0	0	1.25	0.88	0.03	0.08	0.86	0	0.14	0.20	2.19
381	**Oxtail** raw	0.14	0	0.59	0.09	3.97	0	0	4.79	0.19	0.12	0	0.09	0	0	0	0.40
382	stewed	0.19	0	0.79	0.13	5.26	0	0	6.37	0.25	0.16	0	0.13	0	0	0	0.54
383	stewed (weighed with fat and bones)	0.07	0	0.30	0.05	2.00	0	0	2.42	0.10	0.06	0	0.05	0	0	0	0.21
384	**Sweetbread, lamb** raw	0	0	0.15	0.08	2.17	0	0	2.40	0.12	0.13	0	0.08	0	0	0	0.33
387	**Tongue, lamb** raw	0	0	0.34	0.16	5.40	0	0	5.90	0.47	0.40	0	0	0	0	0	0.87
388	**sheep** stewed	0	0	0.56	0.27	8.87	0	0	9.70	0.77	0.65	0	0	0	0	0	1.42
391	**Tripe** dressed	0	0.02	0.04	0.03	0.67	0	0	0.76	0.03	0.01	0	0	0	0	0	0.04
392	stewed	0	0.04	0.08	0.05	1.20	0	0	1.37	0.05	0.02	0	0	0	0	0	0.07

Fatty acids (g per 100 g food)

No	Food	Saturated												Total
		4:0	6:0	8:0	10:0	12:0	14:0	15:0	16:0	17:0	18:0	20:0	22:0	
	Meat products and dishes													
	Canned meats													
393	**Beef, corned**	0	0	0	0	0	0.36	0.07	3.04	0.14	1.47	0	0	5.08
394	**Ham**	0	0	0	0	0	0.07	0	1.24	0	0.55	0	0	1.86
395	**Ham and pork** chopped	0	0	0	0	0	0.35	0	5.50	0	2.75	0	0	8.60
396	**Luncheon meat**	0	0	0	0	0	0.48	0	6.69	0.08	2.88	0	0	10.13
397	**Stewed steak with** gravy	0	0	0	0	0	0.37	0.07	3.14	0.14	1.52	0	0	5.24
	Offal products													
404	**Liver sausage**	0	0	0	0	0	0.34	0	5.47	0	2.65	0	0	8.46
	Sausages													
405	**Frankfurters**	0	0	0	0	0	0.37	0	6.31	0	3.22	0	0	9.90
407	**Salami**	0	0	0	0	0	0.67	0	11.42	0	5.81	0	0	17.90
408	**Sausages, beef** raw	0	0	0	0	0	0.83	0	5.86	0.11	3.40	0	0	10.20
410	grilled	0	0	0	0	0	0.59	0	4.20	0.08	2.44	0	0	7.31
411	**Sausages, pork** raw	0	0	0	0	0	0.58	0	7.89	0	4.16	0	0	12.63
413	grilled	0	0	0	0	0	0.45	0	6.05	0	3.19	0	0	9.69

No	Food	Mono-unsaturated								Polyunsaturated							
		14:1	15:1	16:1	17:1	18:1	20:1	22:1	Total	18:2	18:3	20:3	20:4	20:5	22:5	22:6	Total
	Meat products and dishes																
	Canned meats																
393	**Beef, corned**	0.17	0	0.71	0.11	4.75	0	0	5.74	0.23	0.15	0	0.11	0	0	0	0.49
394	**Ham**	0	0	0.18	0	2.11	0.03	0	2.32	0.45	0	0	0.04	0	0	0	0.49
395	**Ham and pork**																
	chopped	0	0	0.75	0	10.03	0.18	0	10.96	2.11	0.11	0	0.07	0	0	0	2.29
396	**Luncheon meat**	0	0	0.95	0.10	11.28	0.28	0	12.61	1.96	0.18	0.03	0.05	0	0.08	0	2.30
397	**Stewed steak with**																
	gravy	0.18	0	0.74	0.12	4.91	0	0	5.95	0.23	0.15	0	0.12	0	0	0	0.50
	Offal products																
404	**Liver sausage**	0	0	0.84	0	9.62	0.17	0	10.63	1.96	0.11	0	0	0	0	0	2.07
	Sausages																
405	**Frankfurters**	0	0	0.79	0	10.21	0.16	0	11.16	1.72	0.21	0	0	0	0	0	1.93
407	**Salami**	0	0	1.43	0	18.45	0.29	0	20.17	3.12	0.38	0	0	0	0	0	3.50
408	**Sausages, beef** raw	0	0	0.96	0.21	10.11	0	0	11.28	0.90	0.25	0	0	0	0	0	1.15
410	grilled	0	0	0.69	0.15	7.25	0	0	8.09	0.64	0.18	0	0	0	0	0	0.82
411	**Sausages, pork** raw	0	0	1.10	0	13.89	0.15	0	15.14	2.36	0.18	0	0	0	0	0	2.54
413	grilled	0	0	0.84	0	10.64	0.12	0	11.60	1.81	0.14	0	0	0	0	0	1.95

Fatty acids (g per 100 g food)

No	Food	Saturated												Total
		4:0	6:0	8:0	10:0	12:0	14:0	15:0	16:0	17:0	18:0	20:0	22:0	
	Meat products and dishes *contd*													
415	**Beefburgers** frozen raw	0	0	0	0	0	0.61	0.12	5.16	0.23	2.49	0	0	8.61
416	fried	0	0	0	0	0	0.52	0.10	4.35	0.19	2.10	0	0	7.26
418	**Meat paste**	0	0	0	0	0	0.17	0	2.83	0	1.44	0	0	4.44
	Meat and pastry products													
422	**Sausage roll** flaky pastry	0	0	0	0	0.03	1.03	0	8.33	0.13	4.29	0.22	0.22	14.25
423	short pastry	0	0	0	0	0.03	0.86	0	7.36	0.10	3.79	0.17	0.17	12.48
424	**Steak and kidney pie** pastry top only	0	0	0	0	0.02	0.58	0.03	4.19	0.13	2.16	0.11	0.11	7.33
425	individual	0	0	0	0	0	0.63	0	5.19	0	2.83	0.12	0.10	8.87
	Cooked dishes													
426	**Beef steak pudding**	0	0	0	0	0	0.37	0.06	3.12	0.13	2.43	Tr	0	6.11
427	**Beef stew**	0	0	0	0	0	0.23	0.04	1.93	0.08	0.92	Tr	0	3.20
428	**Bolognese sauce**	0	0	0	0	0	0.21	0.03	2.19	0.07	0.86	0.01	0	3.37
429	**Curried meat**	0	Tr	0.08	0.07	0.49	0.29	0.02	1.66	0.03	0.53	0.03	0	3.20
430	**Hot pot**	0	0	0	0	0	0.13	0.02	1.06	0.05	0.51	0	0	1.77
431	**Irish stew**	0	0	0	0	0	0.37	0.04	1.65	0.07	1.43	0	0	3.56
432	**Irish stew** (weighed with bones)	0	0	0	0	0	0.34	0.04	1.52	0.06	1.31	0	0	3.27
433	**Moussaka**	0.08	0.05	0.03	0.07	0.09	0.46	0.06	2.73	0.08	1.03	0.02	0	4.70
434	**Shepherd's pie**	Tr	Tr	Tr	Tr	0.01	0.23	0.03	1.44	0.06	0.67	0.03	0.03	2.50

No	Food	Mono-unsaturated								Polyunsaturated							
		14:1	15:1	16:1	17:1	18:1	20:1	22:1	Total	18:2	18:3	20:3	20:4	20:5	22:5	22:6	Total
	Meat products and dishes contd																
415	**Beefburgers** frozen																
	raw	0.29	0	1.21	0.19	8.05	0	0	9.74	0.38	0.25	0	0.19	0	0	0	0.82
416	fried	0.24	0	1.02	0.16	6.79	0	0	8.21	0.32	0.21	0	0.16	0	0	0	0.69
418	**Meat paste**	0	0	0.35	0	4.57	0.07	0	4.99	0.77	0.09	0	0	0	0	0	0.86
422	**Sausage roll**																
	flaky pastry	0	0	1.32	0	12.37	1.07	0.95	15.71	2.59	0.20	0	0.15	0.63	(0.22)	(0.21)	4.00
423	short pastry	0	0	1.15	0	11.13	0.85	0.74	13.87	2.35	0.18	0	0.12	0.49	(0.17)	(0.17)	3.48
424	**Steak and kidney pie**																
	pastry top only	0.07	Tr	0.77	0.05	5.92	0.51	0.47	7.79	1.01	0.13	0	0.13	0.31	(0.11)	(0.10)	1.79
425	individual	0	0	0.67	0	7.54	0.26	0.22	8.69	2.02	0.18	0	0	0	0	0	2.20
426	**Beef steak pudding**	0.06	0.04	0.42	0.16	4.21	0	0	4.89	0.26	0.06	0	0.04	0	0	0	0.36
427	**Beef stew**	0.11	0	0.44	0.07	2.99	0	0	3.61	0.22	0.10	0	0.07	0	0	0	0.39
428	**Bolognese sauce**	0.09	0	0.38	0.06	3.78	Tr	Tr	4.31	2.36	0.15	0	0.06	0	0	0	2.57
429	**Curried meat**	0.04	0	0.20	0.03	2.92	0.01	0.01	3.21	2.88	0.13	0	0.03	0	0	0	3.04
430	**Hot pot**	0.06	0	0.25	0.04	1.65	0	0	2.00	0.08	0.05	0	0.04	0	0	0	0.17
431	**Irish stew**	0	0	0.09	0.07	2.61	0	0	2.77	0.17	0.17	0	0	0	0	0	0.34
432	**Irish stew** (weighed with bones)	0	0	0.08	0.06	2.39	0	0	2.53	0.16	0.16	0	0	0	0	0	0.32
433	**Moussaka**	0.10	0.02	0.38	0.07	4.34	0.01	0.01	4.93	2.87	0.19	0	0.05	0	0	Tr	3.11
434	**Shepherd's pie**	0.07	Tr	0.35	0.04	2.11	0.11	0.12	2.80	0.15	0.06	0	0.06	0.08	(0.03)	(0.02)	0.40

Fish and fish products

Fatty acids (g per 100 g food)

No	Food	Saturated									Mono-unsaturated						
		12:0	14:0	15:0	16:0	17:0	18:0	20:0	22:0	Total	14:1	16:1	17:1	18:1	20:1	22:1	Total
	White fish																
438	**Cod** raw, fresh fillets	0	Tr	Tr	0.11	0	0.02	0	0	0.13	0	0.01	0	0.05	Tr	Tr	0.06
439	frozen steaks	0	Tr	Tr	0.09	0	0.01	0	0	0.10	0	Tr	0	0.05	Tr	Tr	0.05
440	baked	0	Tr	Tr	0.18	0	0.03	0	0	0.21	0	0.02	0	0.09	0.02	Tr	0.13
441	baked (weighed with bones and skin)	0	Tr	Tr	0.15	0	0.02	0	0	0.17	0	0.02	0	0.08	0.01	Tr	0.11
443	grilled	0	Tr	Tr	0.20	0	0.03	0	0	0.23	0	0.02	0	0.10	0.02	Tr	0.14
444	poached	0	Tr	Tr	0.17	0	0.03	0	0	0.20	0	0.02	0	0.08	0.01	Tr	0.11
445	poached (weighed with bones and skin)	0	Tr	Tr	0.15	0	0.02	0	0	0.17	0	0.02	0	0.08	0.01	Tr	0.11
446	steamed	0	Tr	Tr	0.14	0	0.02	0	0	0.16	0	0.01	0	0.07	0.01	Tr	0.09
447	steamed (weighed with bones and skin)	0	Tr	Tr	0.11	0	0.02	0	0	0.13	0	0.01	0	0.05	Tr	Tr	0.06
448	**smoked** raw	0	Tr	Tr	0.09	0	0.01	0	0	0.10	0	Tr	0	0.05	Tr	Tr	0.05
449	poached	0	0.01	Tr	0.24	0	0.04	0	0	0.29	0	0.03	0	0.12	0.02	Tr	0.17
450	**dried** salt, boiled	0	Tr	Tr	0.14	0	0.02	0	0	0.16	0	0.01	0	0.07	0.01	Tr	0.09
451	**Haddock, fresh** raw	0	Tr	Tr	0.08	Tr	0.03	0	0	0.11	0	0.02	0	0.06	0.01	Tr	0.09
454	steamed	0	Tr	Tr	0.11	Tr	0.03	0	0	0.14	0	0.02	0	0.08	0.01	Tr	0.11
455	steamed (weighed with bones and skin)	0	Tr	Tr	0.08	Tr	0.03	0	0	0.11	0	0.02	0	0.06	0.01	Tr	0.09
456	**smoked** steamed	0	Tr	Tr	0.13	Tr	0.04	0	0	0.17	0	0.03	0	0.09	0.02	Tr	0.14
457	steamed (weighed with bones and skin)	0	Tr	Tr	0.08	Tr	0.03	0	0	0.11	0	0.02	0	0.06	0.01	Tr	0.09

Fish and fish products *continued*

Fatty acids (g per 100 g food)

No	Food	Polyunsaturated															
		16:2	18:2	20:2	22:2	18:3	20:3	22:3	16:4	18:4	20:4	22:4	20:5	22:5	22:6	24:6	Total
	White fish																
438	**Cod** raw, fresh fillets	0	Tr	0	0	Tr	0	0	0	Tr	0.02	0	0.08	Tr	0.16	0	0.26
439	frozen steaks	0	Tr	0	0	Tr	0	0	0	Tr	0.02	0	0.07	Tr	0.14	0	0.23
440	baked	0	Tr	0	0	Tr	0	0	0	Tr	0.03	0	0.14	0.01	0.28	0	0.46
441	baked (weighed with bones and skin)	0	Tr	0	0	Tr	0	0	0	Tr	0.03	0	0.12	0.01	0.23	0	0.39
443	grilled	0	Tr	0	0	Tr	0	0	0	Tr	0.04	0	0.16	0.01	0.30	0	0.51
444	poached	0	Tr	0	0	Tr	0	0	0	Tr	0.03	0	0.13	0.01	0.26	0	0.43
445	poached (weighed with bones and skin)	0	Tr	0	0	Tr	0	0	0	Tr	0.03	0	0.12	0.01	0.23	0	0.39
446	steamed	0	Tr	0	0	Tr	0	0	0	Tr	0.02	0	0.11	Tr	0.21	0	0.34
447	steamed (weighed with bones and skin)	0	Tr	0	0	Tr	0	0	0	Tr	0.02	0	0.08	Tr	0.16	0	0.26
448	**smoked** raw	0	Tr	0	0	Tr	0	0	0	Tr	0.02	0	0.07	Tr	0.14	0	0.23
449	poached	0	Tr	0	0	Tr	0	0	0	Tr	0.04	0	0.19	0.02	0.37	0	0.62
450	**dried** salt, boiled	0	Tr	0	0	Tr	0	0	0	Tr	0.02	0	0.11	Tr	0.21	0	0.34
451	**Haddock, fresh** raw	0	Tr	0	0	Tr	0	0	0	Tr	0.01	Tr	0.05	0.01	0.10	0	0.17
454	steamed	0	0.01	0	0	Tr	0	0	0	Tr	0.02	0.01	0.07	0.01	0.14	0	0.26
455	steamed (weighed with bones and skin)	0	Tr	0	0	Tr	0	0	0	Tr	0.01	Tr	0.05	0.01	0.10	0	0.17
456	**smoked** steamed	0	0.01	0	0	Tr	0	0	0	Tr	0.02	0.01	0.08	0.02	0.15	0	0.29
457	steamed (weighed with bones and skin)	0	Tr	0	0	Tr	0	0	0	Tr	0.01	Tr	0.05	0.01	0.10	0	0.17

Fish *continued*

Fatty acids (g per 100 g food)

No	Food	Saturated									Mono-unsaturated						
		12:0	14:0	15:0	16:0	17:0	18:0	20:0	22:0	Total	14:1	16:1	17:1	18:1	20:1	22:1	Total
	White fish *contd*																
458	**Halibut** raw	0	0.05	Tr	0.17	0.01	0.04	0	0	0.27	0	0.14	Tr	0.29	0.10	0	0.53
459	steamed	0	0.08	Tr	0.29	0.02	0.07	0	0	0.46	0	0.23	0.01	0.49	0.17	0	0.90
460	steamed (weighed with bones and skin)	0	0.06	Tr	0.22	0.02	0.05	0	0	0.35	0	0.17	0.01	0.37	0.13	0	0.68
461	**Lemon sole** raw	0	0.03	Tr	0.12	Tr	0.03	0	0	0.18	0	0.08	0.02	0.13	0.05	0.01	0.29
464	steamed	0	0.02	Tr	0.08	Tr	0.02	0	0	0.12	0	0.05	0.01	0.08	0.03	Tr	0.17
465	steamed (weighed with bones and skin)	0	0.01	Tr	0.05	Tr	0.01	0	0	0.07	0	0.03	Tr	0.06	0.02	Tr	0.11
466	**Plaice** raw	0	0.05	Tr	0.25	Tr	0.04	0	0	0.34	0	0.23	0.02	0.28	0.06	0.03	0.62
469	steamed	0	0.05	Tr	0.22	Tr	0.03	0	0	0.30	0	0.20	0.01	0.24	0.05	0.03	0.53
470	steamed (weighed with bones and skin)	0	0.02	Tr	0.11	Tr	0.02	0	0	0.15	0	0.10	Tr	0.13	0.03	0.02	0.28
471	**Saithe** raw	0	Tr	Tr	0.03	Tr	0.02	0	0	0.05	0	0.01	Tr	0.07	0.02	0.02	0.12
472	steamed	0	Tr	Tr	0.04	Tr	0.02	0	0	0.06	0	0.02	Tr	0.09	0.02	0.03	0.16
473	steamed (weighed with bones and skin)	0	Tr	Tr	0.03	Tr	0.02	0	0	0.05	0	0.01	Tr	0.07	0.02	0.02	0.12
477	**Whiting** steamed	0	0.02	Tr	0.08	Tr	0.02	0	0	0.12	0	0.03	Tr	0.13	0.05	0.04	0.25
478	steamed (weighed with bones)	0	0.01	Tr	0.06	Tr	0.02	0	0	0.09	0	0.02	Tr	0.09	0.03	0.03	0.17

Fatty acids (g per 100 g food)

No	Food	Polyunsaturated															
		16:2	18:2	20:2	22:2	18:3	20:3	22:3	16:4	18:4	20:4	22:4	20:5	22:5	22:6	24:6	Total
	White fish _contd_																
458	**Halibut** raw	0	0.03	Tr	0	0.06	0	0	0	0.03	0.14	0.04	0.17	0.08	0.25	0	0.80
459	steamed	0	0.04	0.01	0	0.10	0	0	0	0.05	0.24	0.06	0.29	0.14	0.42	0	1.35
460	steamed (weighed with bones and skin)	0	0.03	0.01	0	0.07	0	0	0	0.04	0.18	0.05	0.22	0.10	0.32	0	1.02
461	**Lemon sole** raw	0	Tr	0	0	Tr	0	0	0	0.02	(0.06)	0	(0.24)	0.03	0.11	0	0.46
464	steamed	0	Tr	0	0	Tr	0	0	0	0.01	(0.04)	0	(0.15)	0.02	0.07	0	0.29
465	steamed (weighed with bones and skin)	0	Tr	0	0	Tr	0	0	0	Tr	(0.03)	0	(0.10)	0.01	0.05	0	0.19
466	**Plaice** raw	0.02	0.01	0	0	0.01	0.01	0	0	0.03	(0.05)	0	(0.20)	0.06	0.16	0	0.55
469	steamed	0.01	Tr	0	0	Tr	Tr	0	0	0.03	(0.04)	0	(0.17)	0.05	0.14	0	0.45
470	steamed (weighed with bones and skin)	Tr	Tr	0	0	Tr	Tr	0	0	0.01	(0.02)	0	(0.09)	0.03	0.07	0	0.22
471	**Saithe** raw	0	Tr	0	0	Tr	0	0	0	0.01	(0.01)	0	(0.04)	Tr	0.09	0	0.14
472	steamed	0	Tr	0	0	Tr	0	0	0	Tr	(0.01)	0	(0.05)	Tr	0.11	0	0.17
473	steamed (weighed with bones and skin)	0	Tr	0	0	Tr	0	0	0	Tr	(0.01)	0	(0.04)	Tr	0.09	0	0.14
477	**Whiting** steamed	0	Tr	0	0	Tr	0	0	0	0.01	(0.02)	0	(0.06)	0.01	0.11	0	0.21
478	steamed (weighed with bones)	0	Tr	0	0	Tr	0	0	0	Tr	(0.01)	0	(0.04)	Tr	0.08	0	0.13

Fish *continued*

Fatty acids (g per 100 g food)

No	Food	Saturated									Mono-unsaturated						
		12:0	14:0	15:0	16:0	17:0	18:0	20:0	22:0	Total	14:1	16:1	17:1	18:1	20:1	22:1	Total
	Fatty fish																
482	**Herring** raw†	0	1.12	0.08	2.28	0.03	0.20	0	0	3.71	0	1.67	0	2.53	2.20	2.90	9.30
485	grilled	0	0.78	0.06	1.60	0.02	0.14	0	0	2.60	0	1.17	0	1.78	1.54	2.04	6.53
486	grilled (weighed with bones)	0	0.53	0.04	1.09	0.02	0.10	0	0	1.78	0	0.79	0	1.20	1.05	1.38	4.42
487	**Bloater** grilled	0	1.05	0.08	2.15	0.03	0.19	0	0	3.50	0	1.57	0	2.38	2.07	2.72	8.74
488	grilled (weighed with bones)	0	0.78	0.06	1.59	0.02	0.14	0	0	2.59	0	1.16	0	1.76	1.53	2.02	6.47
489	**Kipper** baked	0	0.69	0.05	1.41	0.02	0.12	0	0	2.29	0	1.03	0	1.56	1.35	1.79	5.73
490	baked (weighed with bones)	0	0.37	0.03	0.76	0.01	0.07	0	0	1.24	0	0.56	0	0.85	0.74	0.97	3.12
491	**Mackerel** raw†	0	0.73	0.07	2.58	0.06	0.51	0	0	3.95	0	0.87	0	2.70	1.04	1.45	6.28
494	**Pilchards** canned in tomato sauce	0	0.42	0	0.98	0	0.31	0	0	1.71	0	0.55	0	0.60	0.05	0.02	1.22
495	**Salmon** raw	0	0.52	0	2.03	0	0.42	0	0	2.97	0	0.65	0	2.46	0.91	0.58	4.60
496	steamed	0	0.56	0	2.20	0	0.46	0	0	3.22	0	0.70	0	2.67	0.98	0.63	4.98
497	steamed (weighed with bones and skin)	0	0.45	0	1.78	0	0.37	0	0	2.60	0	0.57	0	2.15	0.79	0.51	4.02
498	canned	0	0.35	0	1.39	0	0.29	0	0	2.03	0	0.44	0	1.68	0.62	0.40	3.14
499	smoked	0	0.19	0	0.76	0	0.16	0	0	1.11	0	0.24	0	0.92	0.34	0.22	1.72
500	**Sardines** canned in oil, fish only	0	0.40	0	1.81	0	0.45	0	0	2.66	0	0.56	0	6.42	0.18	0.26	7.42
501	canned fish plus oil	0	0.83	0	3.76	0	0.94	0	0	5.53	0	1.16	0	13.36	0.38	0.54	15.44
502	canned in tomato sauce	0	0.54	0	2.20	0	0.52	0	0	3.26	0	0.65	0	2.38	0.15	0.05	3.23
508	**Tuna** canned in oil	0	0	0	3.57	0	0.36	0	0	3.93	0	0	0	8.57	0	0	8.57

a Also contains 0.22 mg 24:1

† See footnote on p 143 of 'The Composition of Foods'

Fish _continued_

Fatty acids (g per 100 g food)

No	Food	Polyunsaturated														
		16:2	18:2	20:2	22:2	18:3	20:3	22:3	16:4	18:4	20:4	22:4	20:5	22:5	22:6	24:6	Total
	Fatty fish																
482	**Herring** raw†	0	0.23	0	0	0.20	0	0	0	0.30	0.10	0	1.17	0.18	1.08	0	3.26
485	grilled	0	0.16	0	0	0.14	0	0	0	0.21	0.07	0	0.82	0.13	0.76	0	2.29
486	grilled (weighed with bones)	0	0.11	0	0	0.10	0	0	0	0.14	0.05	0	0.55	0.09	0.51	0	1.55
487	**Bloater** grilled	0	0.22	0	0	0.19	0	0	0	0.28	0.09	0	1.10	0.17	1.02	0	3.07
488	grilled (weighed with bones)	0	0.16	0	0	0.14	0	0	0	0.21	0.07	0	0.81	0.13	0.75	0	2.27
489	**Kipper** baked	0	0.14	0	0	0.12	0	0	0	0.18	0.06	0	0.72	0.11	0.67	0	2.00
490	baked (weighed with bones)	0	0.08	0	0	0.07	0	0	0	0.10	0.03	0	0.39	0.06	0.36	0	1.09
491	**Mackerel** raw†	0.10	0.23	0	0	0.16	0	0	0	0.28	0.15	0	1.07	0.23	1.85	0	4.07
494	**Pilchards** canned in tomato sauce	0.25	0.06	0	0	0.03	0.04	0	0	0.07	0.03	0	1.04	0.12	0.20	0	1.84
495	**Salmon** raw	0.06	0.15	0	0	0.09	0.15	0	0	0.18	0.05	0	0.89	0.29	1.19	0	3.05
496	steamed	0.07	0.16	0	0	0.09	0.16	0	0	0.20	0.06	0	0.96	0.32	1.29	0	3.31
497	steamed (weighed with bones and skin)	0.06	0.13	0	0	0.08	0.13	0	0	0.16	0.05	0	0.77	0.26	1.04	0	2.68
498	canned	0.04	0.10	0	0	0.06	0.10	0	0	0.13	0.04	0	0.61	0.20	0.81	0	2.09
499	smoked	0.02	0.06	0	0	0.03	0.06	0	0	0.07	0.02	0	0.33	0.11	0.45	0	1.15
500	**Sardines** canned in oil, fish only	0.10	0.96	0	0	0.13	0	0	0	0.14	0	0	0.71	0.09	0.56	0	2.69
501	fish plus oil	0.22	1.99	0	0	0.27	0	0	0	0.30	0	0	1.48	0.19	1.16	0	5.61
502	canned in tomato sauce	0.11	0.69	0	0	0.18	0.08	0	0	0.26	0	0	0.99	0.14	1.28	0	3.73
508	**Tuna** canned in oil	0	7.65	0	0	0.19	0	0	0	0	0	0	0	0	0.17	0	8.01

†See footnote on p 143 of 'The Composition of Foods'

Fish *continued*

Fatty acids (g per 100 g food)

No	Food	Saturated									Mono-unsaturated						
		12:0	14:0	15:0	16:0	17:0	18:0	20:0	22:0	Total	14:1	16:1	17:1	18:1	20:1	22:1	Total
	Crustacea																
518	**Crab** boiled	0	0.05	0.03	0.33	0.04	0.16	0	0	0.61	0	0.18	0	0.55	0.13	0.14	1.00
519	boiled (weighed with shell)	0	Tr	Tr	0.06	Tr	0.03	0	0	0.09	0	0.04	0	0.11	0.02	0.03	0.20
520	canned	0	Tr	Tr	0.06	Tr	0.03	0	0	0.09	0	0.03	0	0.09	0.02	0.02	0.16
521	**Lobster** boiled	0	0.03	0.02	0.22	0.03	0.10	0	0	0.40	0	0.12	0	0.36	0.08	0.09	0.65
522	boiled (weighed with shell)	0	0.01	Tr	0.08	0.01	0.04	0	0	0.14	0	0.04	0	0.13	0.03	0.03	0.23
523	**Prawns** boiled	0	0.02	Tr	0.12	0.02	0.05	0	0	0.21	0	0.06	0	0.19	0.04	0.05	0.34
524	boiled (weighed with shell)	0	Tr	Tr	0.05	Tr	0.02	0	0	0.07	0	0.02	0	0.07	0.02	0.02	0.13
527	**Shrimps** boiled	0	0.04	0.01	0.27	Tr	0.04	0	0	0.36	0	0.10	0.02	0.32	0.04	0.03	0.51
528	boiled (weighed with shell)	0	0.01	Tr	0.09	Tr	0.01	0	0	0.11	0	0.03	Tr	0.11	0.01	Tr	0.15
529	canned	0	0.02	Tr	0.13	Tr	0.02	0	0	0.17	0	0.05	Tr	0.16	0.02	0.01	0.24
	Molluscs																
532	**Mussels** raw[a]	0	0.03	0.01	0.16	0.02	0.10	0	0	0.33	0	0.09	0	0.09	0.10	0.07	0.35
533	boiled[b]	0	0.04	0.01	0.17	0.02	0.10	0	0	0.36	0	0.09	0	0.10	0.11	0.07	0.37
534	boiled (weighed with shell)	0	0.01	Tr	0.05	Tr	0.03	0	0	0.09	0	0.03	0	0.03	0.03	0.02	0.11
535	**Oysters** raw	0	0.03	Tr	0.13	0.01	0.03	0	0	0.20	0	0.02	0	0.04	0.02	0.02	0.10
536	raw (weighed with shell)	0	Tr	Tr	0.01	Tr	Tr	0	0	0.01	0	Tr	0	Tr	Tr	Tr	0.00
538	**Scallops** steamed[c]	0.05	0.04	0.01	0.17	Tr	0.04	0	0	0.34	0.02	0.04	0	0.05	0.03	0.02	0.14
	Fish products and dishes																
548	**Fish pie**[d]	0.06	0.38	0.02	1.15	0.05	0.45	0.08	0.07	2.40	0.02	0.26	0.02	1.24	0.32	0.33	2.19
549	**Kedgeree**	0.01	0.24	Tr	1.43	0.05	0.52	0.08	0.08	2.41	0	0.33	0	1.77	0.36	0.36	2.82
550	**Roe, cod** hard, raw	0	0.02	Tr	0.26	Tr	0.02	0	0	0.30	0	0.08	0	0.23	0.02	Tr	0.33

[a] Also contains 0.01 mg 24:0 [b] Also contains 0.02 mg 24:0 [c] Also contains 0.03 mg 13:0
[d] Also contains 0.05 mg 4:0; 0.03 mg 6:0; 0.02 mg 8:0 and 0.04 mg 10:0

Fish continued

Fatty acids (g per 100 g food)

Polyunsaturated

No	Food	16:2	18:2	20:2	22:2	18:3	20:3	22:3	16:4	18:4	20:4	22:4	20:5	22:5	22:6	24:6	Total
	Crustacea																
518	**Crab** boiled	0.11	0.12	0.09	0	0.17	0	0.06	0	0.08	0.02	0.04	0.78	0.05	0.37	0.04	1.93
519	boiled (weighed with																
	shell)	0.02	0.02	0.02	0	0.03	0	0.01	0	0.02	Tr	Tr	0.15	Tr	0.07	Tr	0.34
520	canned	0.02	0.02	0.02	0	0.03	0	0.01	0	0.01	Tr	Tr	0.14	Tr	0.06	Tr	0.31
521	**Lobster** boiled	0.07	0.08	0.06	0	0.11	0	0.04	0	0.05	0.01	0.03	0.51	0.03	0.24	0.02	1.25
522	boiled (weighed with																
	shell)	0.02	0.03	0.02	0	0.04	0	0.01	0	0.02	Tr	Tr	0.18	0.01	0.09	Tr	0.42
523	**Prawns** boiled	0.04	0.04	0.03	0	0.06	0	0.02	0	0.03	Tr	0.01	0.27	0.02	0.13	0.01	0.66
524	boiled (weighed with																
	shell)	0.01	0.02	0.01	0	0.02	0	Tr	0	0.01	Tr	Tr	0.11	Tr	0.05	Tr	0.23
527	**Shrimps** boiled	0	0.02	0	0	0.02	0	0.03	0	0.02	0.02	0.02	0.36	0.02	0.26	0	0.77
528	boiled (weighed with																
	shell)	0	Tr	0	0	Tr	0	Tr	0	Tr	Tr	Tr	0.12	Tr	0.09	0	0.21
529	canned	0	0.01	0	0	0.01	0	0.01	0	Tr	0.01	Tr	0.18	0.01	0.13	0	0.36
	Molluscs																
532	**Mussels** raw[a]	0.02	0.03	0.02	0.02	0.02	0	0.01	0.01	0.07	0.06	0	0.15	0.03	0.06	0	0.52
533	boiled[a]	0.03	0.03	0.02	0.02	0.02	0	0.01	0.01	0.08	0.06	0	0.16	0.03	0.06	0	0.55
534	boiled (weighed with																
	shell)	Tr	Tr	Tr	Tr	Tr	0	Tr	Tr	0.02	0.02	0.01	0.05	Tr	0.02	0	0.11
535	**Oysters** raw	0	0.01	0	0	Tr	0	0	0	0.03	0.01	0.01	0.10	0.01	0.11	0	0.28
536	raw (weighed with																
	shell)	0	Tr	0	0	Tr	0	0	0	Tr	Tr	Tr	0.01	Tr	0.01	0	0.02
538	**Scallops** steamed	0.02	Tr	0	0.01	0.01	0	0.03	0	0.03	0.04	0	0.11	Tr	0.08	0	0.33
	Fish products and dishes																
548	**Fish pie**	0	0.27	0	0	0.03	0	0	0	0	0.05	0	0.24	0.08	0.12	0	0.79
549	**Kedgeree**	0	0.44	0	0	Tr	0	0	0	Tr	0.08	Tr	0.27	0.08	0.17	0	1.04
550	**Roe, cod** hard, raw	0	Tr	0	0	Tr	0	0	0	Tr	0.04	0	0.20	0.02	0.28	0	0.54

[a] Also contains 0.02 mg 19:3

Vegetables

Fatty acids (g per 100 g food)

No	Food	Saturated											Total
		4:0	6:0	8:0	10:0	12:0	14:0	15:0	16:0	17:0	18:0	20:0	22:0	Total
562	**Beans, runner** raw	0	0	0	0	0	0	0	0.03	0	Tr	0	0	0.03
563	boiled	0	0	0	0	0	0	0	0.03	0	Tr	0	0	0.03
569	**baked** canned in tomato sauce	0	0	0	0	0	0	0	0.08	0	Tr	0	0	0.08
597	**Cucumber** raw	0	0	0	0	Tr	Tr	0	0.03	0	Tr	0	0	0.03
609	**Mushrooms** raw	0	0	0	0	0	Tr	0	0.13	0	Tr	0	0	0.13
620	**Peas, fresh** raw	0	0	0	0	0	Tr	0	0.10	0	0.05	0	0	0.15
621	boiled	0	0	0	0	0	Tr	0	0.10	0	0.05	0	0	0.15
622	**frozen** raw	0	0	0	0	0	Tr	0	0.10	0	0.05	0	0	0.15
623	boiled	0	0	0	0	0	Tr	0	0.10	0	0.05	0	0	0.15
624	**canned** garden	0	0	0	0	0	Tr	0	0.07	0	0.04	0	0	0.11
625	processed	0	0	0	0	0	Tr	0	0.10	0	0.05	0	0	0.15
626	**dried** raw	0	0	0	0	0	0.02	0	0.31	0	0.15	0	0	0.48
627	boiled	0	0	0	0	0	Tr	0	0.10	0	0.05	0	0	0.15
628	**split** dried, raw	0	0	0	0	0	0.02	0	0.24	0	0.12	0	0	0.38
629	boiled	0	0	0	0	0	Tr	0	0.07	0	0.04	0	0	0.11
634	**Peppers, green** raw	0	0	0	0	Tr	Tr	0	0.05	0	0.01	Tr	0	0.06
635	boiled	0	0	0	0	Tr	Tr	0	0.05	0	0.01	Tr	0	0.06
639	**Potatoes, old** raw	0	0	0	0	0	0	0	0.01	0	Tr	0	0	0.01
640	boiled	0	0	0	0	0	0	0	0.01	0	Tr	0	0	0.01
642	baked	0	0	0	0	0	0	0	0.01	0	Tr	0	0	0.01
643	baked (weighed with skins)	0	0	0	0	0	0	0	0.01	0	Tr	0	0	0.01

Fatty acids (g per 100 g food)

No	Fcod	Mono-unsaturated								Polyunsaturated						
		14:1	15:1	16:1	17:1	18:1	20:1	22:1	Total	18:2	18:3	20:4	20:5	22:5	22:6	Total
562	**Beans, runner** raw	0	0	Tr	0	Tr	0	0	0.00	0.05	0.06	0	0	0	0	0.11
563	boiled	0	0	Tr	0	Tr	0	0	0.00	0.05	0.06	0	0	0	0	0.11
569	**baked** canned in tomato sauce	0	0	0	0	0.05	0	0	0.05	0.10	0.15	0	0	0	0	0.25
597	**Cucumber** raw	0	0	Tr	0	Tr	0	0	0.00	0.02	0.02	0	0	0	0	0.04
609	**Mushrooms** raw	0	0	Tr	0	Tr	0	0	0.00	0.06	0.27	0	0	0	0	0.33
620	**Peas, fresh** raw	0	0	Tr	0	0.12	Tr	0	0.12	0.03	Tr	0	0	0	0	0.03
621	boiled	0	0	Tr	0	0.12	Tr	0	0.12	0.03	Tr	0	0	0	0	0.03
622	**frozen** raw	0	0	Tr	0	0.12	Tr	0	0.12	0.03	Tr	0	0	0	0	0.03
623	boiled	0	0	Tr	0	0.12	Tr	0	0.12	0.03	Tr	0	0	0	0	0.03
624	**canned** garden	0	0	Tr	0	0.09	Tr	0	0.09	0.03	Tr	0	0	0	0	0.03
625	processed	0	0	Tr	0	0.12	Tr	0	0.12	0.03	Tr	0	0	0	0	0.03
626	**dried** raw	0	0	0.03	0	0.38	Tr	0	0.41	0.11	0.03	0	0	0	0	0.14
627	boiled	0	0	Tr	0	0.12	Tr	0	0.12	0.03	Tr	0	0	0	0	0.03
628	**split** dried, raw	0	0	0.02	0	0.29	Tr	0	0.31	0.09	0.02	0	0	0	0	0.11
629	boiled	0	0	Tr	0	0.09	Tr	0	0.09	0.03	Tr	0	0	0	0	0.03
634	**Peppers, green** raw	0	0	Tr	0	0.02	0	0	0.02	0.18	0.04	0	0	0	0	0.22
635	boiled	0	0	Tr	0	0.02	0	0	0.02	0.18	0.04	0	0	0	0	0.22
639	**Potatoes, old** raw	0	0	Tr	0	Tr	0	0	0.00	0.05	0.01	0	0	0	0	0.06
640	boiled	0	0	Tr	0	Tr	0	0	0.00	0.05	0.01	0	0	0	0	0.06
642	baked	0	0	Tr	0	Tr	0	0	0.00	0.05	0.01	0	0	0	0	0.06
643	baked (weighed with skins)	0	0	Tr	0	Tr	0	0	0.00	0.05	0.01	0	0	0	0	0.06

Vegetables *continued*

Fatty acids (g per 100 g food)

No	Food	Saturated												Total
		4:0	6:0	8:0	10:0	12:0	14:0	15:0	16:0	17:0	18:0	20:0	22:0	
	Potatoes *contd*													
648	**new** boiled	0	0	0	0	0	0	0	0.01	0	Tr	0	0	0.01
649	canned	0	0	0	0	0	0	0	0.01	0	Tr	0	0	0.01
650	**instant** powder	0	0	0	0	0	0	0	0.11	0	0.03	0	0	0.14
651	made up	0	0	0	0	0	0	0	0.03	0	Tr	0	0	0.03
657	**Spinach** boiled	0	0	0	0	0	Tr	0	0.05	0	0.01	0	0	0.06
661	**Sweetcorn, on-the-cob** raw	0	0	0	0	0	0.01	0	0.32	0	0.05	Tr	0	0.38
662	boiled	0	0	0	0	0	0.01	0	0.31	0	0.05	Tr	0	0.37
663	**canned** kernels	0	0	0	0	0	Tr	0	0.07	0	0.01	Tr	0	0.08
664	**Sweet potatoes** raw	0	0	0	Tr	0.03	Tr	0	0.17	Tr	0.02	Tr	0	0.22
665	boiled	0	0	0	Tr	0.03	Tr	0	0.17	Tr	0.02	Tr	0	0.22
669	**Turnips** raw	0	0	0	0	0	0	0	0.03	0	Tr	0	0	0.03
670	boiled	0	0	0	0	0	0	0	0.03	0	Tr	0	0	0.03

Vegetables *continued*

No	Food	Mono-unsaturated								Polyunsaturated						
		14:1	15:1	16:1	17:1	18:1	20:1	22:1	Total	18:2	18:3	20:4	20:5	22:5	22:6	Total
	Potatoes contd															
648	**new** boiled	0	0	Tr	0	Tr	0	0	0.00	0.05	0.01	0	0	0	0	0.06
649	canned	0	0	Tr	0	Tr	0	0	0.00	0.05	0.01	0	0	0	0	0.06
650	**instant** powder	0	0	Tr	0	0.01	0	0	0.01	0.36	0.11	0	0	0	0	0.47
651	made up	0	0	Tr	0	Tr	0	0	0.00	0.09	0.03	0	0	0	0	0.12
657	**Spinach** boiled	0	0	Tr	0	0.03	0	0	0.03	0.05	0.25	0	0	0	0	0.30
661	**Sweetcorn, on-the-cob** raw	0	0	Tr	0	0.69	Tr	Tr	0.69	1.15	0.04	0	0	0	0	1.19
662	boiled	0	0	Tr	0	0.66	Tr	Tr	0.66	1.10	0.04	0	0	0	0	1.14
663	**canned** kernels	0	0	Tr	0	0.14	Tr	Tr	0.14	0.24	Tr	0	0	0	0	0.24
664	**Sweet potatoes** raw	0	0	Tr	0	0.03	0	0	0.03	0.16	0.03	0	0	0	0	0.19
665	boiled	0	0	Tr	0	0.03	0	0	0.03	0.16	0.03	0	0	0	0	0.19
669	**Turnips** raw	0	0	Tr	Tr	0.02	0	0	0.02	0.04	0.14	0	0	0	0	0.18
670	boiled	0	0	Tr	Tr	0.02	0	0	0.02	0.04	0.14	0	0	0	0	0.18

Fatty acids (g per 100 g food)

No	Food	Saturated												Total
		4:0	6:0	8:0	10:0	12:0	14:0	15:0	16:0	17:0	18:0	20:0	22:0	
692	**Avocado pears**†	0	0	0	0	0	0	0	2.61	0	0	0	0	2.61
693	**Bananas** raw	0	0	0	0	0	0	0	0.10	0	Tr	0	0	0.10
694	raw weighed with skins	0	0	0	0	0	0	0	0.07	0	Tr	0	0	0.07
771	**Olives** in brine	0	0	0	0	0	0	0	1.26	0	0.24	0.04	0	1.54
772	in brine (weighed with stones)	0	0	0	0	0	0	0	1.01	0	0.19	0.03	0	1.23

†The fat content varies according to season

Fruit

No	Food	Mono-unsaturated								Polyunsaturated						
		14:1	15:1	16:1	17:1	18:1	20:1	22:	Total	18:2	18:3	20:4	20:5	22:5	22:6	Total
692	**Avocado pears**†	0	0	0.74	0	15.94	0	0	16.68	1.83	0.08	0.02	0	0	0	1.93
693	**Bananas** raw	0	0	Tr	0	0.03	0	0	0.03	0.04	0.05	0	0	0	0	0.09
694	raw weighed with skins	0	0	Tr	0	0.02	0	0	0.02	0.03	0.03	0	0	0	0	0.06
771	**Olives** in brine	0	0	0.11	0	7.57	0	0	7.68	1.16	0.07	0	0	0	0	1.23
772	in brine (weighed with stones)	0	0	0.08	0	6.06	0	0	6.14	0.93	0.06	0	0	0	0	0.99

†The fat content varies according to season

Fatty acids (g per 100 g food)

No	Food	Saturated													Total
		4:0	6:0	8:0	10:0	12:0	14:0	15:0	16:0	17:0	18:0	20:0	22:0	24:0	
822	**Almonds**	0	0	0	0	0	0.05	0	3.22	0	0.87	0.10	0	0	4.24
823	(weighed with shells)	0	0	0	0	0	0.02	0	1.19	0	0.32	0.04	0	0	1.57
824	**Barcelona nuts**	0	0	0	0	0	0.18	0	3.18	0	1.10	0.12	0	0	4.58
825	(weighed with shells)	0	0	0	0	0	0.11	0	1.97	0	0.68	0.08	0	0	2.84
826	**Brazil nuts**	0	0	0	0	0	0.12	0	9.17	0	6.41	0	0	0	15.70
827	(weighed with shells)	0	0	0	0	0	0.05	0	4.12	0	2.88	0	0	0	7.05
828	**Chestnuts**	0	0	0	0	0	0	0	0.43	0	0.03	0.01	0	0	0.47
829	(weighed with shells)	0	0	0	0	0	0	0	0.35	0	0.02	0.01	0	0	0.38
830	**Cob or hazel nuts**	0	0	0	0	0	0.10	0	1.79	0	0.62	0.07	0	0	2.58
831	(weighed with shells)	0	0	0	0	0	0.04	0	0.65	0	0.22	0.02	0	0	0.93
832	**Coconut** fresh	0	0.24	2.54	2.41	16.18	5.36	0	3.05	0	0.81	0.34	0	0	30.93
834	desiccated	0	0.41	4.38	4.15	27.86	9.23	0	5.26	0	1.40	0.58	0	0	53.27
835	**Peanuts** fresh	0	0	0	0	0.05	0.23	0	5.01	0	1.26	0.56	1.59	0.52	9.22
836	(weighed with shells)	0	0	0	0	0.03	0.16	0	3.46	0	0.87	0.39	1.10	0.36	6.37
837	roasted and salted	0	0	0	0	0.05	0.23	0	5.01	0	1.26	0.56	1.59	0.52	9.22
838	**Peanut butter** smooth	0	0	0	0	0	0	0	5.80	0	2.82	0.72	1.28	0	10.62
839	**Walnuts**	0	0	0	0	0	0.54	0	3.69	0	1.03	0.34	0	0	5.60
840	(weighed with shells)	0	0	0	0	0	0.35	0	2.37	0	0.66	0.22	0	0	3.60

Fatty acids (g per 100 g food)

No	Food	Mono-unsaturated								Polyunsaturated						
		14:1	15:1	16:1	17:1	18:1	20:1	22:1	Total	18:2	18:3	20:4	20:5	22:5	22:6	Total
822	**Almonds**	0	0	0.36	0	36.26	0	0	36.62	9.77	0.26	0	0	0	0	10.03
823	(weighed with shells)	0	0	0.13	0	13.42	0	0	13.55	3.62	0.09	0	0	0	0	3.71
824	**Barcelona nuts**	0	0	0.18	0	49.38	0.06	0	49.62	6.55	0.12	0	0	0	0	6.67
825	(weighed with shells)	0	0	0.11	0	30.55	0.04	0	30.70	4.05	0.08	0	0	0	0	4.13
826	**Brazil nuts**	0	0	0.24	0	19.93	0	0	20.17	22.93	0	0	0	0	0	22.93
827	(weighed with shells)	0	0	0.11	0	8.94	0	0	9.05	10.29	0	0	0	0	0	10.29
828	**Chestnuts**	0	0	0.02	0	0.99	0	0	1.01	0.97	0.11	0	0	0	0	1.08
829	(weighed with shells)	0	0	0.01	0	0.81	0	0	0.82	0.79	0.09	0	0	0	0	0.88
830	**Cob or hazel nuts**	0	0	0.10	0	27.77	0.03	0	27.90	3.68	0.07	0	0	0	0	3.75
831	(weighed with shells)	0	0	0.04	0	10.03	0.01	0	10.08	1.33	0.02	0	0	0	0	1.35
832	**Coconut** fresh	0	0	0.14	0	2.24	0	0	2.38	0.61	0	0	0	0	0	0.61
834	desiccated	0	0	0.23	0	3.85	0	0	4.08	1.05	0	0	0	0	0	1.05
835	**Peanuts** fresh	0	0	0	0	22.95	0.52	0	23.47	13.58	0.37	0	0	0	0	13.95
836	(weighed with shells)	0	0	0	0	15.83	0.36	0	16.19	9.37	0.26	0	0	0	0	9.63
837	roasted and salted	0	0	0	0	22.95	0.52	0	23.47	13.58	0.37	0	0	0	0	13.95
838	**Peanut butter** smooth	0	0	0	0	26.49	0.72	0	27.21	13.45	0	0	0	0	0	13.45
839	**Walnuts**	0	0	0.10	0	7.93	0	0	8.03	29.54	5.61	0	0	0	0	35.15
840	(weighed with shells)	0	0	0.06	0	5.08	0	0	5.14	18.93	3.60	0	0	0	0	22.53

Sugars and preserves, confectionery and beverages

Fatty acids (g per 100 g food)

No	Food	Saturated																Total
		4:0	6:0	8:0	10:0	12:0	14:0	15:0	16:0	17:0	18:0	20:0	22:0					
	Sugars and preserves																	
852	**Lemon curd** home made	0.32	0.20	0.12	0.28	0.35	1.13	0.11	3.29	0.10	1.35	0	0					7.25
854	**Marzipan** almond paste	0	0	0	0	0	0.02	0	1.50	0	0.40	0.05	0					1.97
	Confectionery																	
857	**Chocolate**, milk	0.14	0.12	0	0.17	0.26	0.98	0	8.12	0	7.71	0.17	0					17.67
858	plain	0	0	0	0	0.14	0.45	0	7.48	0	9.18	0.14	0					17.39
	Beverages																	
868	**Cocoa powder**	0	0	0	0	0	0	0	5.44	0	7.16	0.19	0					12.79
873	**Drinking chocolate**	0	0	0	0	0	0.03	0	1.53	0	1.92	0.05	0					3.53
	Alcoholic beverages																	
916	**Advocaat**	0	0	0	0	0	Tr	0	1.50	0	0.49	0	0					1.99

Sugars and preserves, confectionery and beverages

No	Food	Mono-unsaturated								Polyunsaturated							
		14:1	15:1	16:1	17:1	18:1	20:1	22:1	Total	18:2	18:3	20:4	20:5	22:5	22:6	22:5& 22:6	Total
	Sugars and preserves																
852	**Lemon curd** home made	0.14	0.07	0.37	0.11	3.81	0	0	4.50	0.40	0.15	0.02	0	0	0.03	0	0.60
854	**Marzipan** almond paste	0	0	0.17	0	16.88	0	0	17.05	4.55	0.12	0	0	0	0	0	4.67
	Confectionery																
857	**Chocolate**, milk	0	0	0.17	0	9.53	0	0	9.70	0.83	0.23	0	0	0	0	0	1.06
858	plain	0	0	0	0	9.38	0	0	9.38	0.92	0	0	0	0	0	0	0.92
	Beverages																
868	**Cocoa powder**	0	0	0	0	7.22	0	0	7.22	0.62	0	0	0	0	0	0	0.62
873	**Drinking chocolate**	0	0	0	0	1.99	0	0	1.99	0.18	0	0	0	0	0	0	0.18
	Alcoholic beverages																
916	**Advocaat**	Tr	0	0.22	0	2.24	0	0	2.46	0.58	Tr	0.04	0	0	0.06	0	0.68

Fatty acids (g per 100 g food)

No	Food	Saturated												
		4:0	6:0	8:0	10:0	12:0	14:0	15:0	16:0	17:0	18:0	20:0	22:0	Total
	Sauces and pickles													
920	**Bread sauce**	0.10	0.06	0.04	0.09	0.11	0.43	0.03	1.13	0.04	0.47	0.03	0.03	2.56
922	**Cheese sauce**	0.29	0.18	0.11	0.25	0.33	1.28	0.10	3.28	0.14	1.38	0.10	0.10	7.54
925	**French dressing**	0	0	0	0	0	0	0	8.37	0	1.61	0.28	0	10.26
927	**Onion sauce**	0.08	0.05	0.03	0.07	0.09	0.47	0.03	1.34	0.06	0.55	0.07	0.07	2.91
933	**Tomato sauce**	0	0	0	0	Tr	0.09	0	0.52	0.01	0.24	0.02	0.02	0.90
934	**White sauce** savoury	0.29	0.18	0.11	0.25	0.33	1.28	0.10	3.27	0.14	1.38	0.10	0.10	7.53
935	sweet	0.12	0.08	0.05	0.11	0.15	0.78	0.04	2.17	0.10	0.90	0.12	0.12	4.74
	Soups													
943	**Lentil**	0.02	0.01	Tr	0.02	0.03	0.23	Tr	0.70	0.03	0.28	0.05	0.05	1.42

Fatty acids (g per 100 g food)

No	Food	Mono-unsaturated								Polyunsaturated							
		14:1	15:1	16:1	17:1	18:1	20:1	22:1	Total	18:2	18:3	20:4	20:5	22:5	22:6	22:5 & 22:6	Total
	Sauces and pickles																
920	**Bread sauce**	0.04	0.02	0.16	0.03	1.20	0.11	0.12	1.68	0.21	0.06	0.02	0.08	N	N	0.05	0.42
922	**Cheese sauce**	0.13	0.06	0.52	0.10	3.54	0.41	0.42	5.18	0.39	0.15	0.06	0.28	N	N	0.19	1.07
925	**French dressing**	0	0	0.70	0	50.25	0	0	50.95	7.68	0.49	0	0	0	0	0	8.17
927	**Onion sauce**	0.03	0.02	0.27	0.03	1.45	0.31	0.32	2.43	0.24	0.04	0.05	0.21	N	N	0.15	0.69
933	**Tomato sauce**	0	0	0.11	0	0.72	0.11	0.11	1.05	0.13	Tr	0.02	0.07	N	N	0.05	0.27
934	**White sauce** savoury	0.13	0.06	0.52	0.10	3.53	0.41	0.42	5.17	0.34	0.14	0.06	0.28	N	N	0.19	1.01
935	sweet	0.05	0.03	0.45	0.04	2.36	0.50	0.52	3.95	0.33	0.07	0.09	0.34	N	N	0.24	1.07
	Soups																
943	**Lentil**	Tr	Tr	0.17	Tr	0.76	0.23	0.24	1.40	0.13	0.01	0.03	0.16	N	N	0.11	0.44

Printed in England for Her Majesty's Stationery Office by Hobbs the Printers of Southampton
(2140) Dd0599386 K12 6/80 G327